I0558462

Sipping with FREEALITEA

Recipes for a Relaxing Escape with Herbal Teas

By Dr. Michelle Clay, DO, CHHC

Table of Contents

Introduction

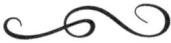

Tea has become an everyday ritual for me in some way shape or form. I have created ways to have a relaxing escape right where I am with herbal teas in my cup or cocktail glass. Whether it is a smoothie in the morning to start my day or a warm tonic at night to wind down after a busy day. As I sip my tea mocktail or cocktail, my mind and soul begin to soothe from the day's worries if only for a moment. Sipping has become a soothing ritual; a way to quench the thirst in my soul not just my palate.

Life seems complicated with the many responsibilities and day to day fires we must put out. It seems like if it's not one thing it's another! But it's simple. Take it moment by moment by creating your me-time moment. Just take a slow breath in, sip and allow every flavor of the tea cascade over each taste bud, exhale, and enjoy the experience. This is sipping for your FREEALITEA – your stress-FREE reality by Sipping with FREEALITEA.

To begin with simplicity, let's start with simple syrups. It's an easy way to have a sweet, savory, and concentrated form of your tea to prepare some of the recipes in this book.

Traditionally a simple syrup is made with equal parts sugar and water. To make it a little healthier, substitute sugar for honey. If sugar is used, only raw cane sugar that has not been processed as much as white granulated sugar is a better option.

Using a simple syrup as a sweetener evenly disperses the sweetness throughout your beverage or whatever dish you choose to use it for. I have used a simple syrup to sweeten my hot tea, as well as make unique salad dressings like the recipes in Cooking for FREEALITEA. Try it for yourself and explore the possibilities.

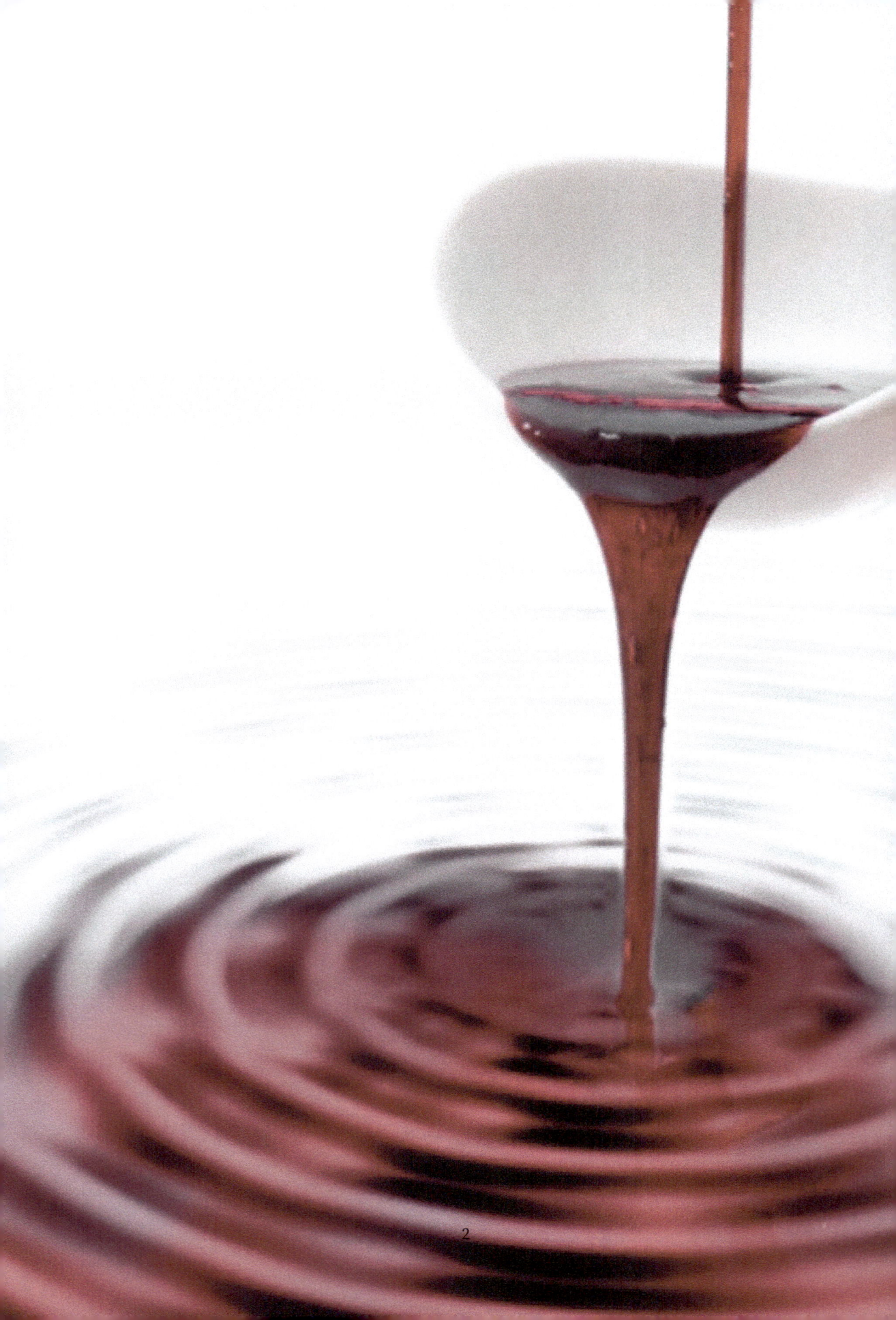

FREEALITEA Simple Syrups

INGREDIENTS

1/3 cup Honey or Raw Cane Sugar

2 tbsp FREEALITEA tea blend

1 ¼ cup Distilled Water

INSTRUCTIONS

- In a medium pot, bring water to a boil. Remove from the heat, add FREEALITEA tea to the pot. Cover and steep 5-7 minutes.

*NOTE you can place tea in a tea bag or diffuser for easier steeping

- Strain and add the honey or cane sugar to the pot of tea. Bring to a boil over high heat. Stir to mix ingredients well until honey or sugar have dissolved.
- Boil 3-5 minutes. Reduce heat and simmer 15 – 20 minutes. You'll begin to see bubbles form then a slight foam.
- Continue heating until the liquid has reached desired thickness but not too thick.
- Allow mixture to cool to room temperature.
- Pour into a mason jar or other airtight glass container and store in the refrigerator.
- Will last for approximately a month.

Chapter 1

Release Recharge

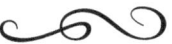

Release Recharge is FREEALITEA's first born. Her formula came to me one day while sitting on my sofa contemplating life and how I could eliminate the loneliness I felt in a house that was supposed to be my home with my fiancé'.

Have you ever been in a house full of people and still felt alone? I knew that my life was not supposed to feel like that. A home is supposed to be a place of refuge and rest, but instead it was stress and strain. It was during this time that a group of herbs came to me: hibiscus, rosemary, juniper berry and others. I didn't know what it was for or why, but I knew it was important, so I wrote them down in my journal. A couple of weeks later during my prayer and meditation time, God directed me to put them together as a tea and see what would happen. I experimented with the ratios of each herb to create a tea. I remember the first time I boiled the water and added about a tablespoon to it to steep. The smell was AMAZING! I anxiously waited for it to steep and cool so I could taste it. With anticipation, I blew into the cup so I wouldn't burn my tongue and took my first sip. "What is this?! I've never tasted anything like this! Second sip, "Mmmmm." Third sip, "ahhhhh", exhale....

With every sip, my mind started to slow down. My shoulders began to relax. My heart felt the warmth of love and by the time I got to the bottom of the mug it felt like my mother just hugged me. Calm, ease, and love washed over me. I had released and felt recharged.

Release Recharge Ingredients:
- Hibiscus flowers
- Rosemary
- Juniper Berries
- Rose Hips
- Cinnamon
- Moringa Leaf
- Alfalfa

Release Recharge Benefits:

- Clinical trials have shown that hibiscus can lower blood pressure and suggest that hibiscus tea may be as potent as some blood pressure medications. Hibiscus also helps lower cholesterol levels and promotes weight loss.

- Rosemary helps lift the mood while relieving stress. It also increases blood flow to the brain which helps improve memory and mood

- Cinnamon helps lower blood sugar by increasing insulin sensitivity. This is helpful for people with type 2 diabetes. Cinnamon improves memory and helps lift mood with smell.

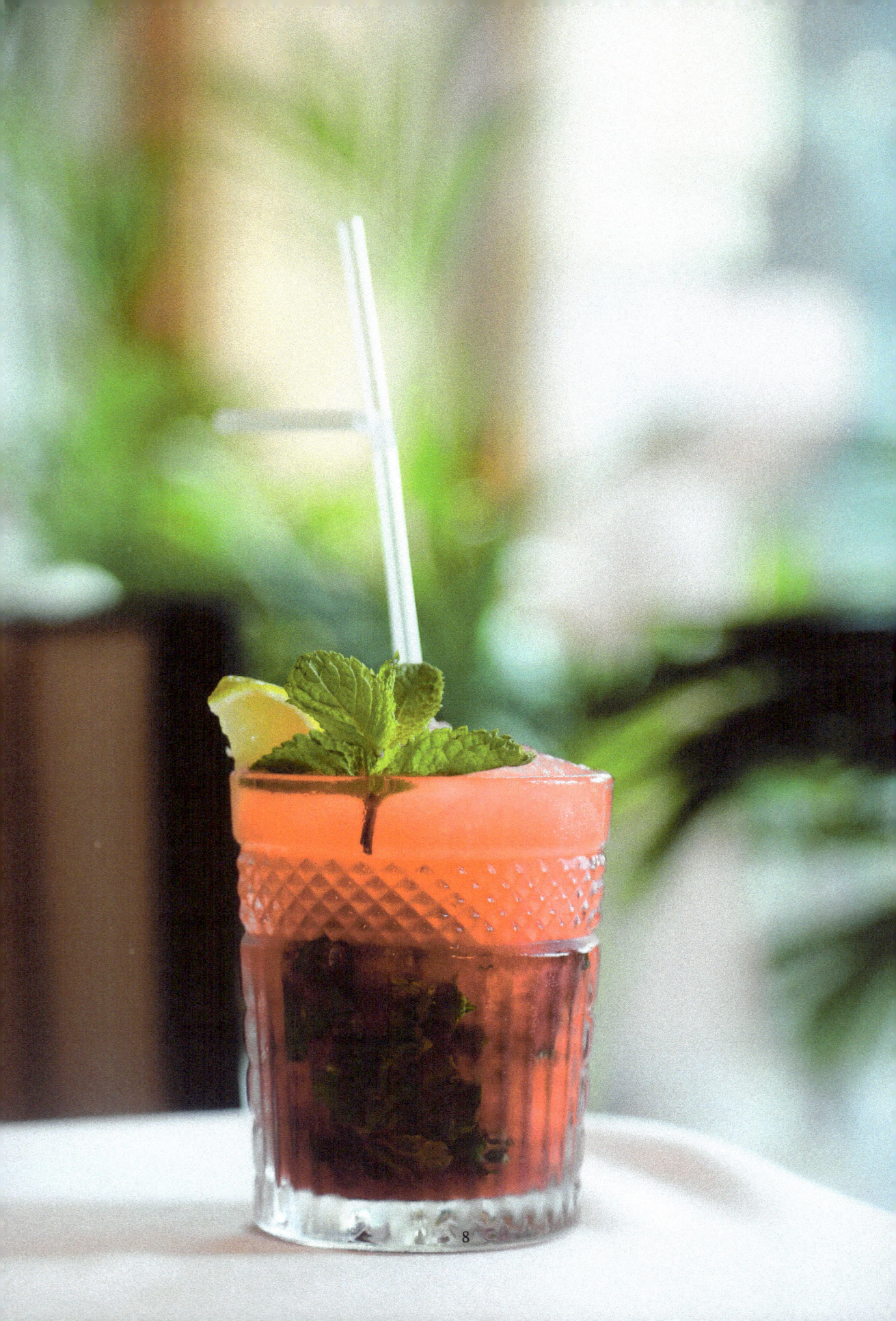

Recharge My Mojo Mojito

INGREDIENTS

2 tbsp. Release Recharge Simple Syrup

5-10 Mint Leaves

1-2 tsp. Cane Sugar

Juice of 1 Lime

2 oz Caribbean Rum

4 oz. Club Soda

Cubed or crushed ice

Lime wedge and mint sprig for garnish (optional)

INSTRUCTIONS

Gently muddle the mint in the bottom of a tall glass (such as a mojito glass, highball).

Note If you don't have a muddler, use a wooden spoon.

Pour in sugar and gently muddle into mint. Add lime juice, rum and Release recharge simple syrup. Stir gently to combine. Fill the glass with ice.

Slowly pour in club soda to fill the glass and gently stir to mix.

**Optional Serve with a garnish of lime and mint

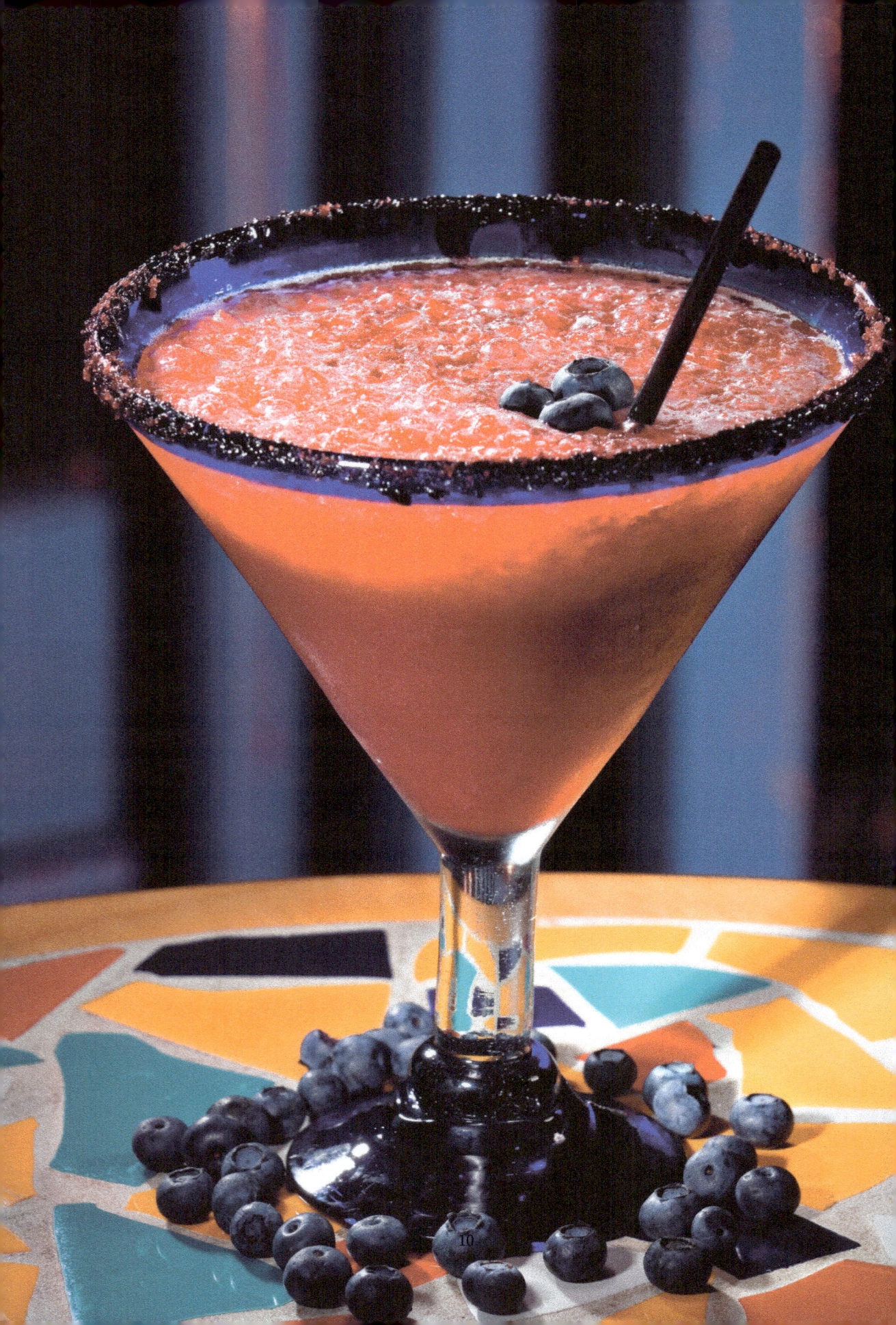

Blueberry Margarita

INGREDIENTS

Release Recharge Simple Syrup

2 cups fresh blueberries

1 lime, juiced

2/3 cup cane sugar or honey

10 ounces silver tequila

8 ounces Grand Marnier

8 ounces lime juice

lime wedges for serving

INSTRUCTIONS

Place the blueberries and juice from 1 lime in a saucepan over low heat. Heat until the blueberries begin to burst and become liquidy and soft. Transfer the mixture to a food processor and blender and puree until smooth.

In a large pitcher, mix the tequila, Grand Marnier, lime juice, blueberry puree and half of the Release Recharge simple syrup. At this point, taste and make adjustments as necessary.

Rim each glass with a lime wedge dip into sugar or salt. Your choice depending on how you like your margaritas. Fill with crushed ice.

Pour the drink over the crushed ice and serve with extra lime wedges.

CHEERS!

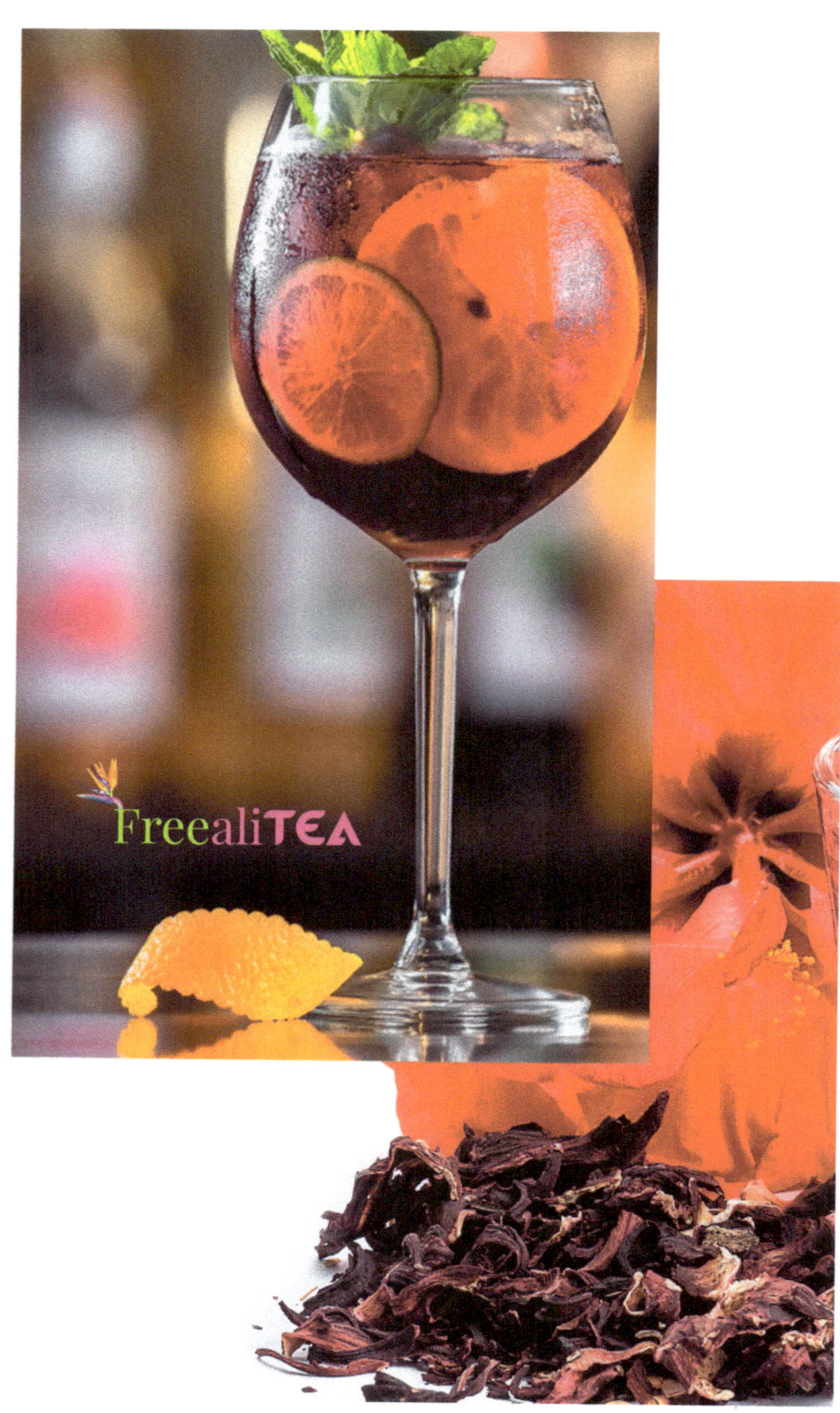

R&R Sangria

FreealiTEA

R&R Sangria

INGREDIENTS

2 oranges, halved and thinly sliced

1 small granny smith apple, core removed and thinly sliced

1 lime, thinly sliced

1-pint raspberries

1-pint blueberries

3 cups of Release Recharge Tea brewed, chilled, and sweetened

½ cup ginger beer

1½ cup red wine

INSTRUCTIONS

Bring 3 ½ cups of water to a boil. Add 3 tablespoons of Release Recharge tea. Allow to steep for at least 10 minutes. Strain and sweeten to taste. Chill in the refrigerator for at least 1 hour.

In a large pitcher, combine oranges, apples, lime slices, and raspberries. Using a wooden spoon, muddle the fruit until there is about ¼ cup of juice

Add Release Recharge tea that has already been brewed,

Stir and mix

Pour into glasses with fruit, about 2/3 full.

Top with ginger beer and serve

Makes 8 servings

*OPTIONAL To enhance the flavor, add a shot of bourbon

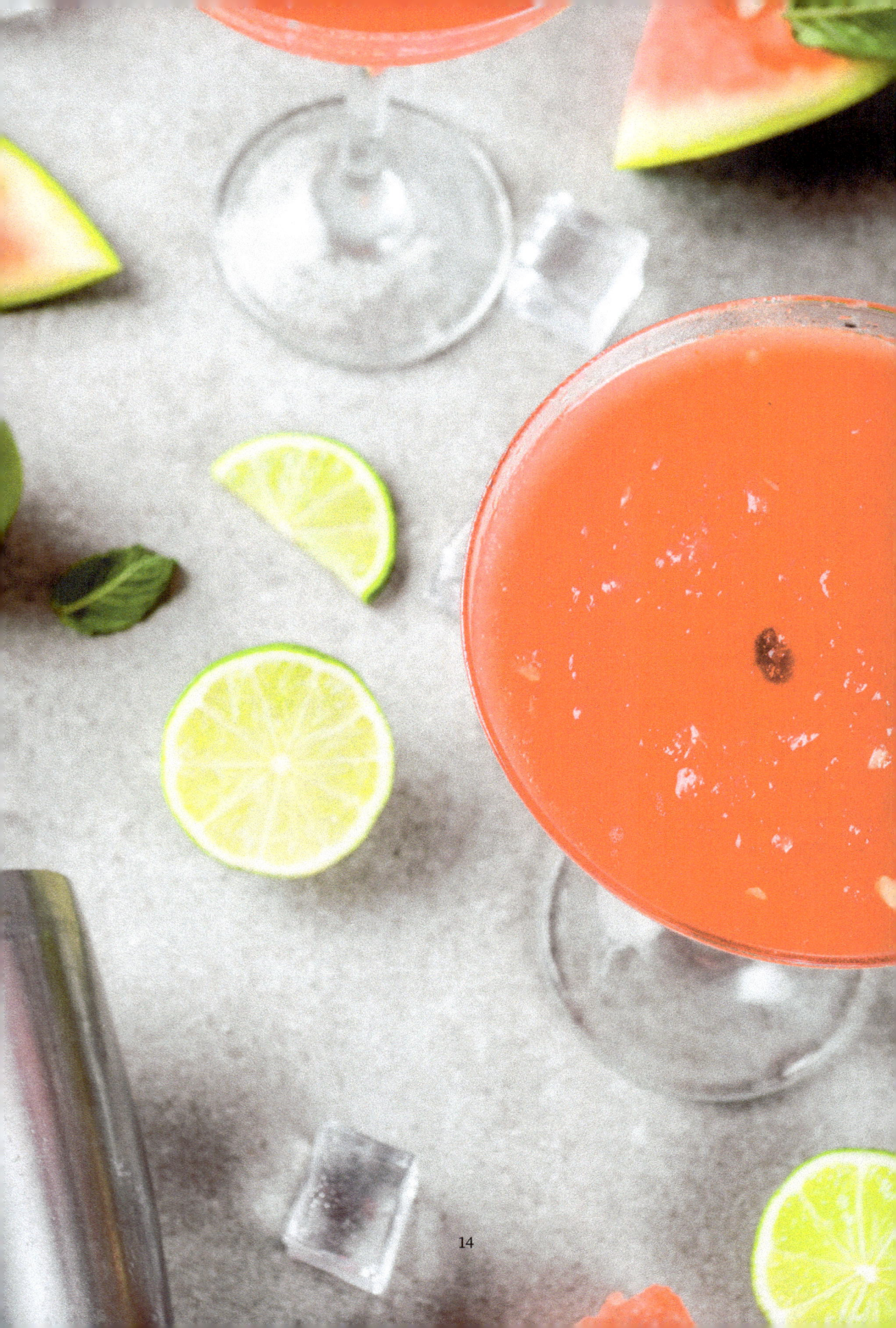

Melon, Mint & Mellow

INGREDIENTS

3 tbsp. Release Recharge simple syrup

1/3 cup of Honey

3 cups of Watermelon

10 Mint leaves (adjust according to taste)

2 oz. Tequila (I personally like Don Julio)

lime wedges for serving

INSTRUCTIONS

Juice watermelon by blending. Once juiced add mint leaves and blend.

Add 2-3 tablespoons of Release Recharge simple syrup and blend.

Divide this mixture between 2 glasses. Add tequila and a squeeze of fresh lime juice.

Stir and enjoy!

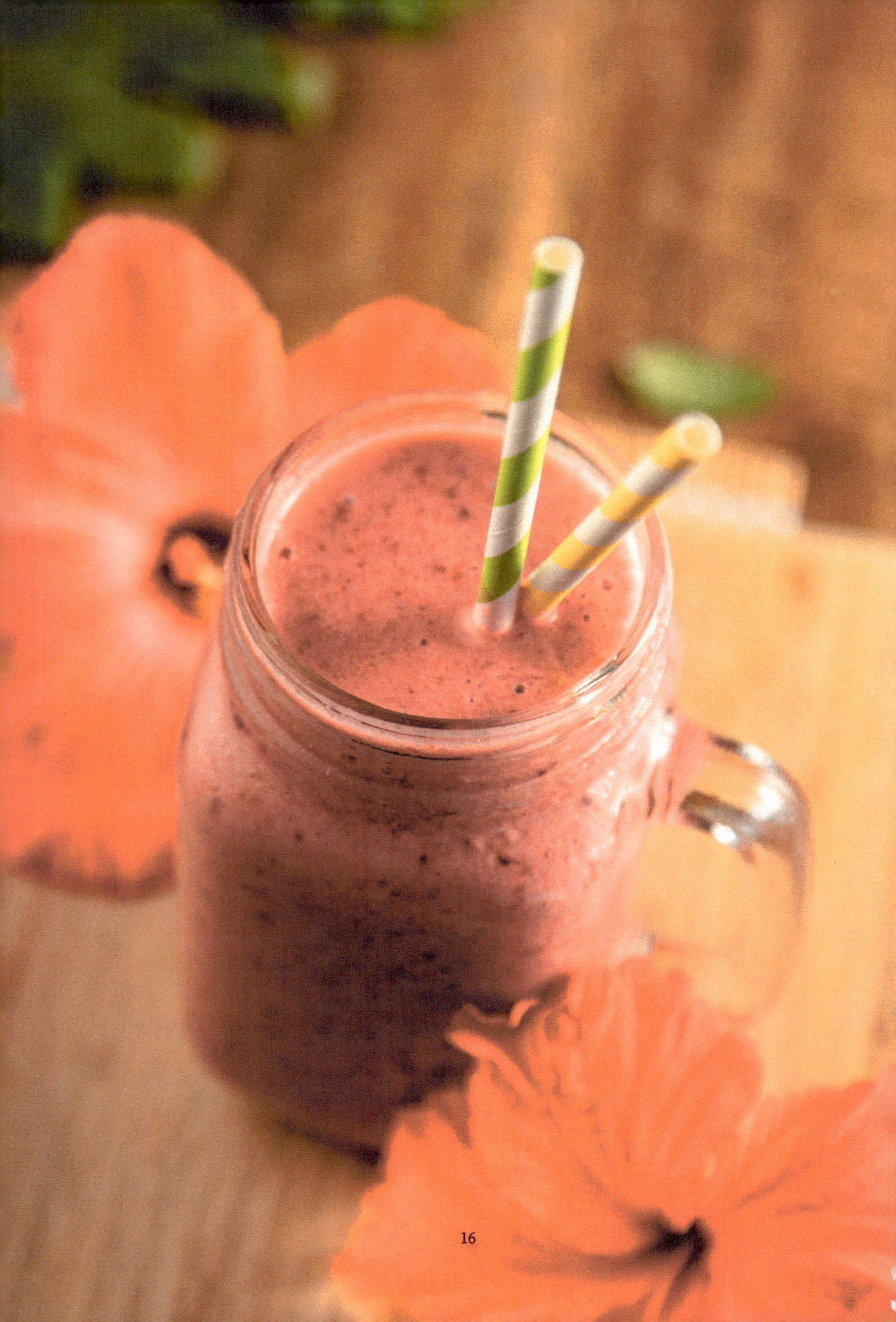

Recharge Citrus Smoothie

INGREDIENTS

1 tbsp. Release Recharge tea

10 oz. Distilled or Spring Water

½ Orange, peeled

Juice of 1 Lime

½ inch of ginger root

Handful of Spinach or Baby Kale

INSTRUCTIONS

Bring water to a boil

Add 1 tablespoon of Release Recharge tea to pot or mug with hot water. (Can add tea to empty tea bags or loose in pan). Let steep for 7-10 minutes.

Using a strainer (or remove tea bags) strain the tea. Sweeten to taste.

Allow to cool. May make ahead of time and chill in the refrigerator until ready for use.

In a blender, combine brewed and chilled Release Recharge tea and lime juice.

Blend. While blender is still running, add ginger root.

Next add orange and spinach or kale.

Blend until smooth.

Pour in a glass and enjoy!

Chapter 2

Release Your RoyalTEA

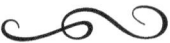

R elease Your RoyalTEA is a very special blend. It was born during a time when my 7 ½ year relationship just ended. Hopes I had for the future of marriage, children, commitment, and contentment were washed away. We lived together for 7 of those years and began planning our wedding, as well as started raising his daughter together. It was A LOT! It was during this time after the separation that I was working to heal and reclaim myself. Have you ever been in a situation where you compromise repeatedly for the benefit of the relationship and your mate's feelings until you are unrecognizable? Yes, that was me. I had to remind myself that I was special. I was beautiful. I was royal! I could picture a beautiful, vibrant purple tea in my mind but didn't know how to make it that color without food coloring. My research led me to butterfly pea flower.

Butterfly pea flower is a flower native to Thailand. It is used as a natural coloring for foods and textiles. The beauty of this flower is not only is it beautiful, but it has calming properties. The anxious feelings I had about my future and wondering if I would ever find that one person that I could build and share a life with dissipated as I sipped this tea.

Drinking Release Your RoyalTEA is like having your own personal affirmation book in a cup. While it is steeping it says, "You are special and unique. No one can do it or be it like you."

Once you begin to sip, it says,   "You are powerful."

"You are phenomenal"

"You are ROYALTY"

Release Your RoyalTEA Ingredients:

- ❧ Purple Leaf Tea
- ❧ Butterfly Pea Flower
- ❧ Ashwagandha
- ❧ Dried Blueberries

Release Your RoyalTEA Benefits:

- Purple leaf tea has more antioxidants than green tea. The antioxidant, anthocyanin which give it its rich purple color helps improve heart health, protect against cancer, reduce pain and inflammation, and boost immunity.
- Ashwagandha is classified as an adaptogen herb. Meaning it helps protect the body from the adverse effects of stress and stress-induced exhaustion. It calms and energizes you at the same time.

The Kama Sutra identifies ashwagandha as a potent igniter of passion and desire. It increases libido, sex drive, and sexual performance.

In traditional Ayurvedic medicine, ashwagandha is known as "the strength of a stallion" and has been used as a sedative, a rejuvenating tonic and anti-inflammatory.

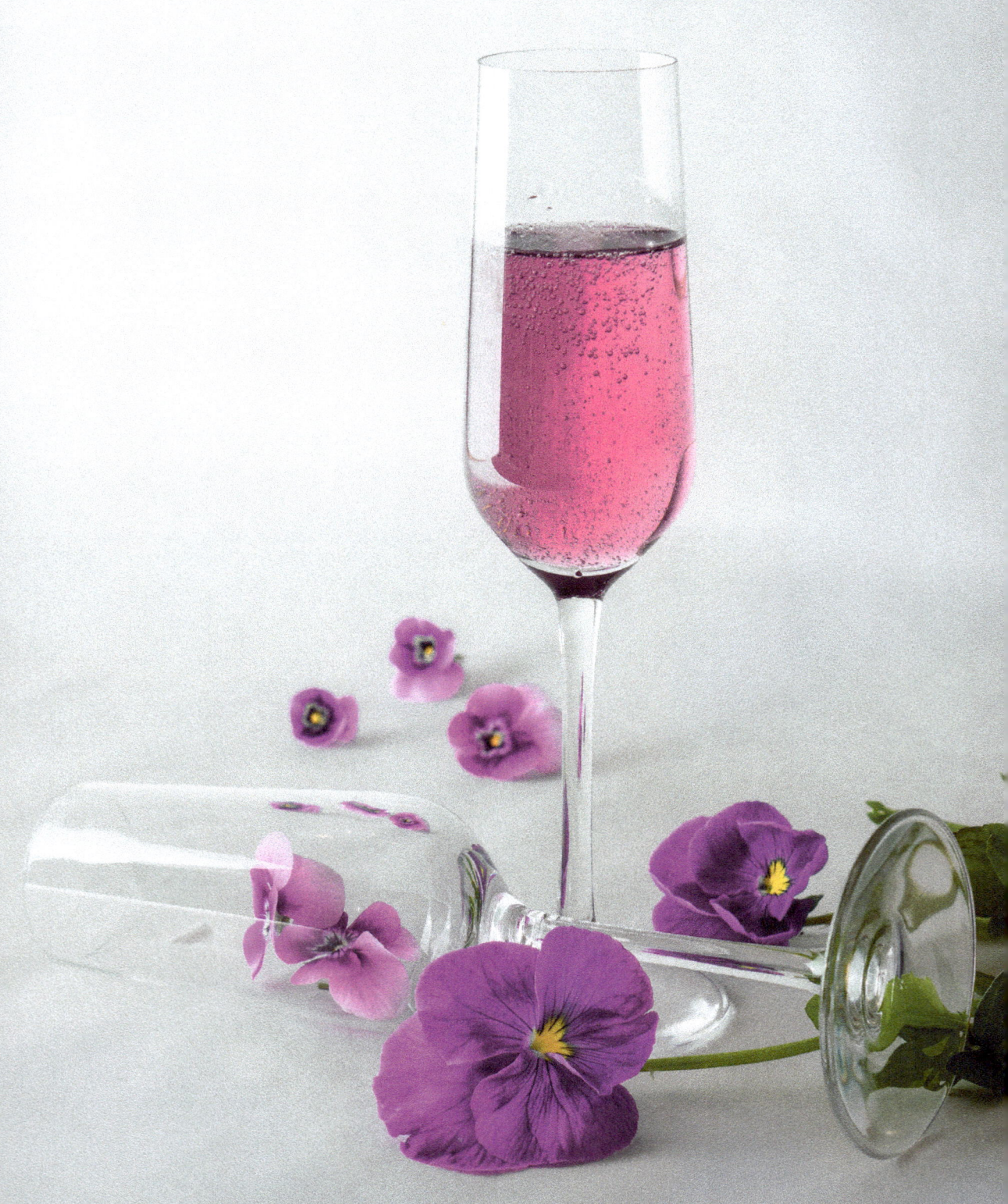

Royale RoyalTEA

INGREDIENTS

½ cup of Release Your RoyalTEA brewed and sweetened if desired

1 oz. Chambord

6 ounces chilled dry Champagne

INSTRUCTIONS

Pour Release Your RoyalTEA to a Champagne flute

Add the Chambord

While holding the glass at a 45-degree angle (this helps preserve the bubbles), gently pour in the Champagne.

Garnish with a raspberry, if desired.

Serve immediately, TOAST and ENJOY!

*NOTES

One bottle of Champagne will make approximately 5 drinks. One small (375 mL) bottle of Chambord is enough for 25 drinks. So, you'll need five times as much Champagne as Chambord.

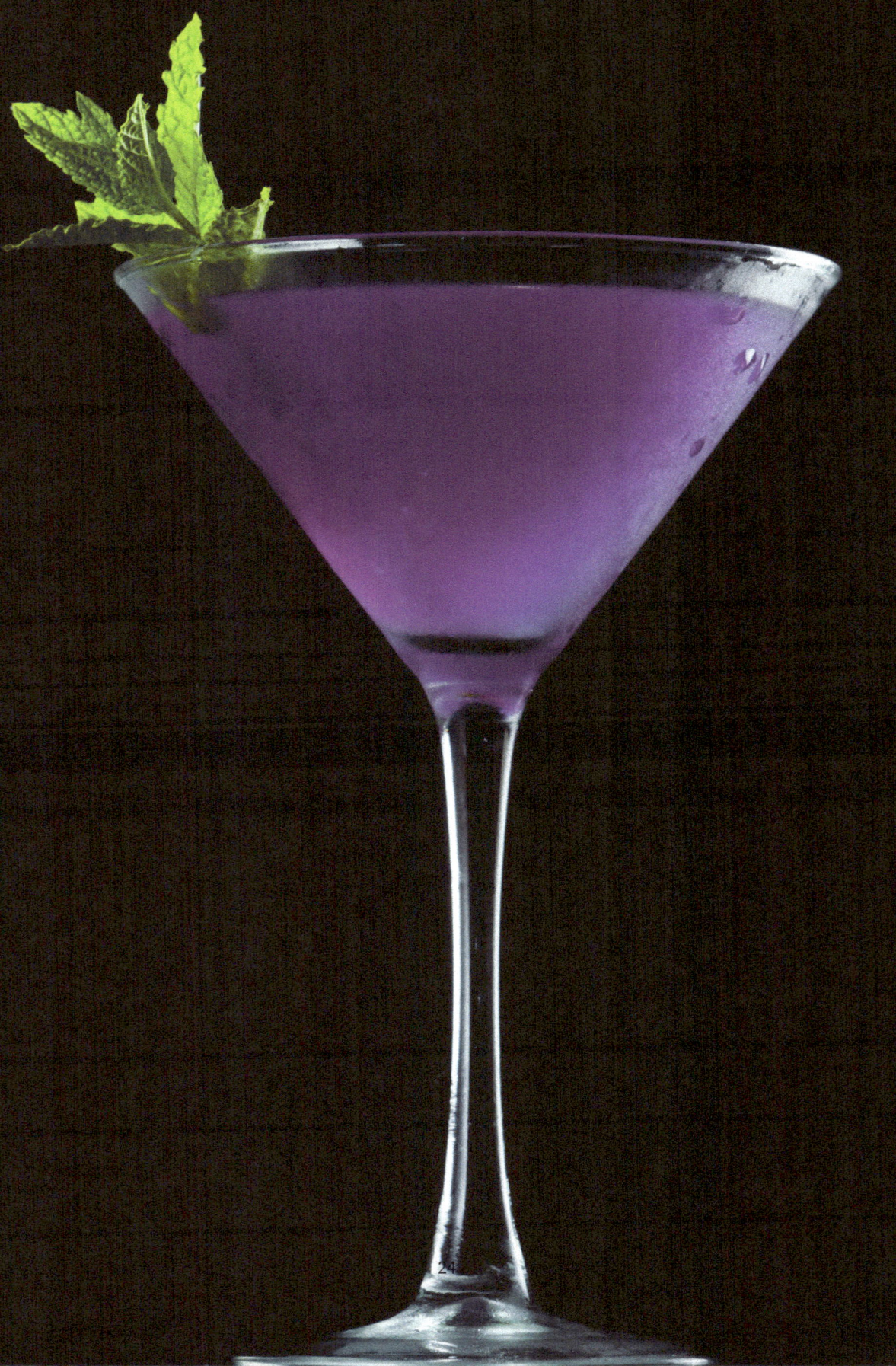

RoyalTEANI

INGREDIENTS

1 cup water

1 tbsp of Release Your RoyalTEA

2 oz. Chambord Liquor optional

2 oz. good quality Vodka. I prefer Grey Goose

Honey

Mint springs, Raspberries, Oranges, etc. for garnish

INSTRUCTIONS

Bring water to a boil. Add 1 tablespoon of Release Your RoyalTEA to pot (can add tea to empty tea bags or loose in pan). Let steep for 7-10 minutes.

Using a strainer (or remove tea bags) strain the tea. Sweeten to taste with honey/ agave etc. Allow to cool. Chill in the refrigerator for at least 1 hour (this can be made ahead of time).

Mix brewed RoyalTEA, Chambord, and vodka in a cocktail shaker.

Pour into ice-filled glasses.

Garnish with a mint sprig, raspberries, oranges, whatever you love.

ENJOY!!

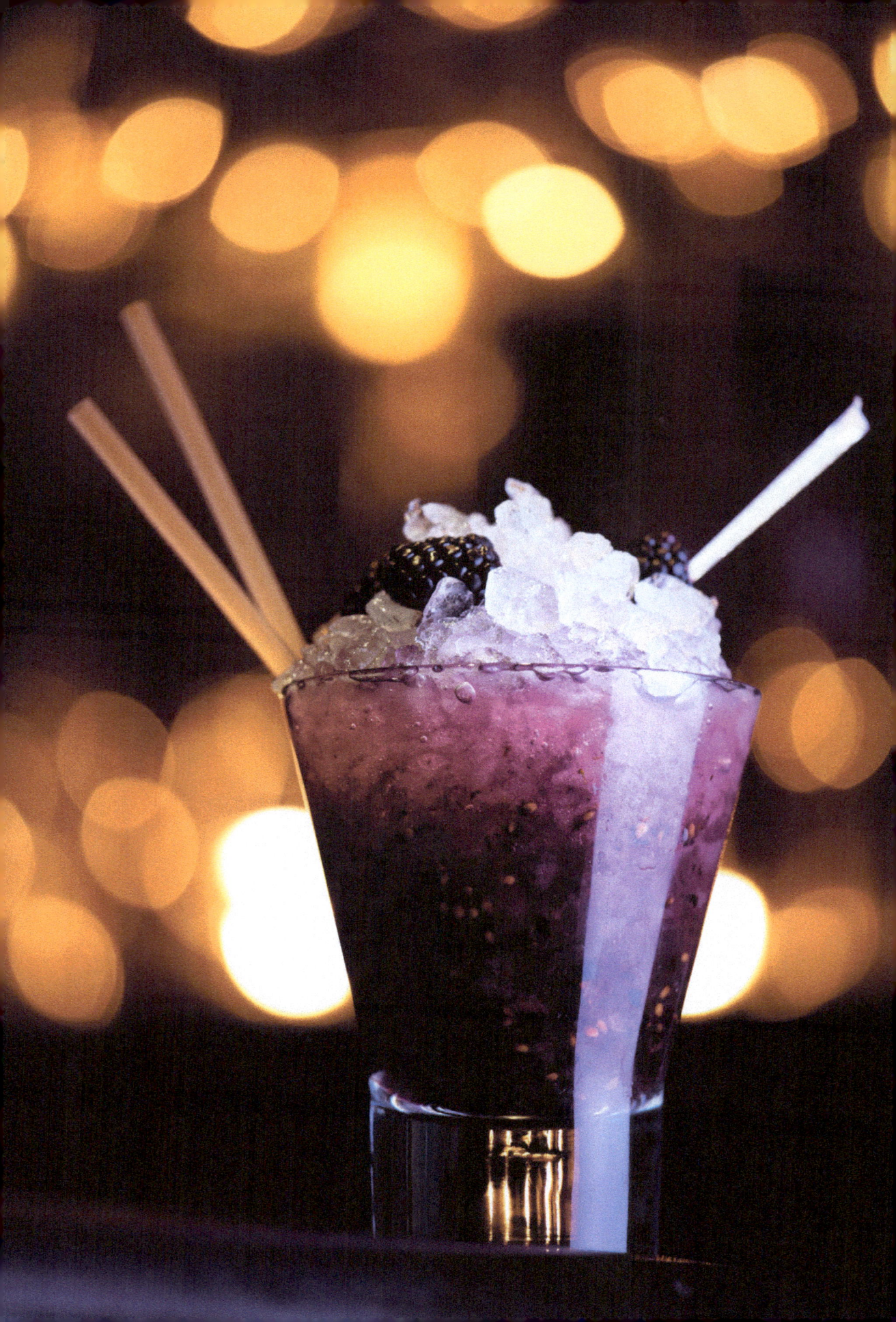

Royal Carnival

Mardi Gras or Carnival season is a time to celebrate life to the fullest. It is an opportunity to "do whatcha wanna" and dance and drink your cares away. There is NO JUDGEMENT during Mardi Gras. You will see anything and EVERYTHING in the street. But it is so much fun! I l always release my inner child and just be free! Because New Orleans doesn't have an open container law, you can go to parties, balls, and parades and bring your special cocktail with you. Not in a glass, but what is called, "a go-cup". Some of the coveted "throws" or items thrown from the parade floats, are signature plastic cups. Perfect to fill and refill as needed to keep the good times rollin'!

This FREEALITEA cocktail is an ode to New Orleans Carnival season.

Laissez Les Bon Temps Rouler!

INGREDIENTS
2 Tbsp of Release Your Royal TEA
2 cups of Spring of Distilled Water
Handful of Blackberries
4 ounces of Gin
Fresh Basil Leaves
Honey or desired sweetener
Juice of 1 Lime

INSTRUCTIONS

Bring water to a boil. Add 2 tablespoons of Release Your RoyalTEA to pot (can add tea to empty tea bags or loose in pan). Let steep for 7-10 minutes.

Using a strainer (or remove tea bags) strain the tea. Sweeten to taste with honey/agave etc.

Allow to cool. Chill in the refrigerator for at least 1 hour (this can be made ahead of time).

In a cocktail shaker, muddle blackberries with gin, basil leaves, and lime juice,

Double strain, using a fine-mesh strainer, to remove seeds.

Add the brewed and chilled Release Your Royal TEA.

Shake well.

Fill 3-4 rock glasses ½ way with ice. Divide cocktail among the glasses.

Garnish with a basil leaf, slice of lime, or blackberry. Or all 3 if you wanna!

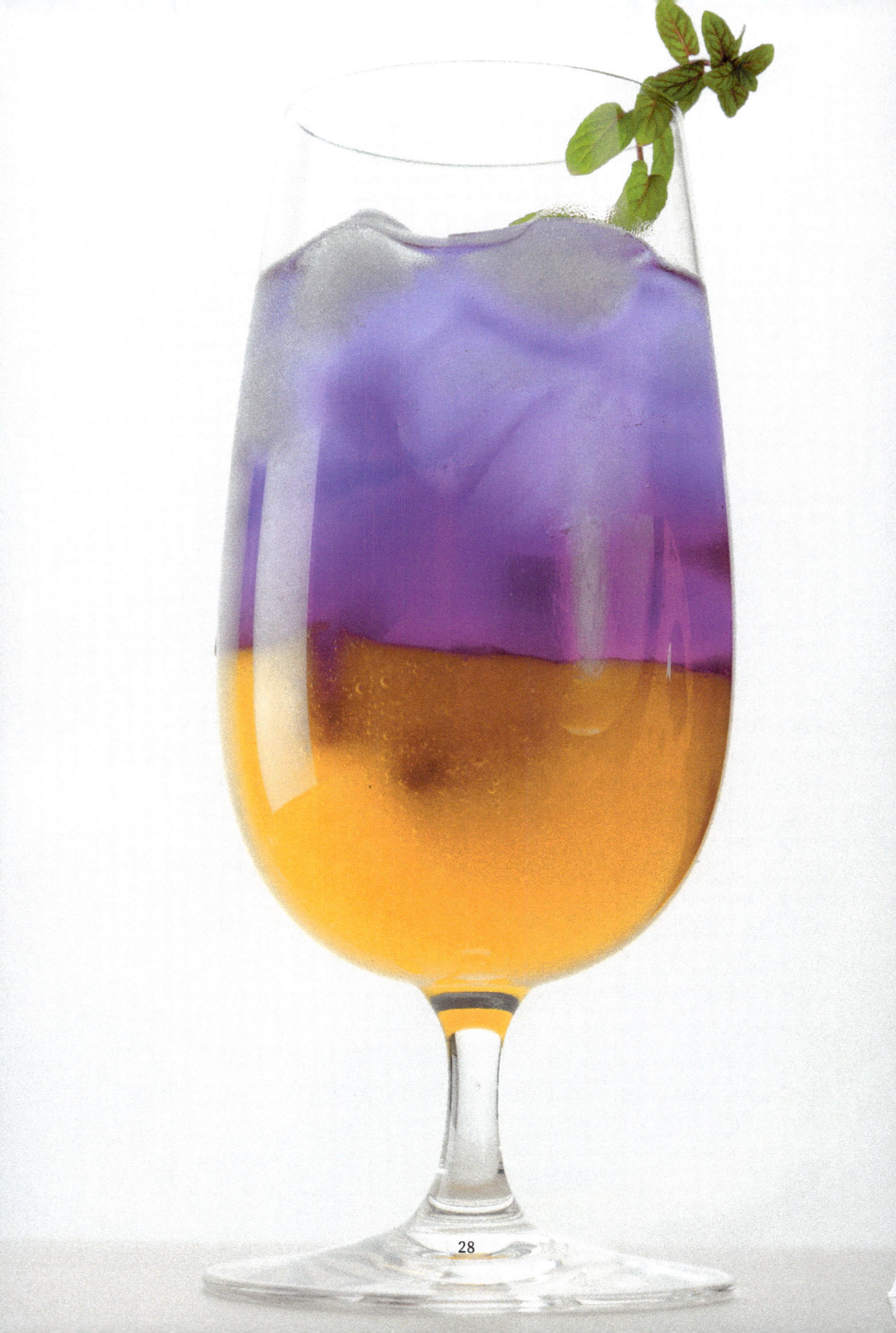

Royal Passion

INGREDIENTS

1 cup water

1 tablespoon Release Your RoyalTEA

½ cup fresh squeezed lime juice

½ cup Passion fruit juice cocktail

Ice

Fresh Mint leaves for garnish optional

INSTRUCTIONS

To brew tea heat water to boiling. Once it has reached a boil, turn off the heat. Add dried Release Your RoyalTEA. Stir, cover and steep for 5-7 minutes.

Strain (or if you placed the tea in a tea bag or diffuser), remove tea. Tea should be a vibrant purple-bluish color. Allow to cool tea for at least 30 minutes.

*NOTE This can be made ahead of time to allow it to completely cool.

In a measuring cup, mix lime juice and passion fruit juice. Stir and pour ¼ cup of the combined liquid into four glasses with ice.

Slowly pour cooled tea on top of mixed juice with ice. Pour very slowly so as not to mix the lower layer and cause a full, immediate color change.

Garnish with mint. Serve with a straw.

***Optional make the G & G version by adding vodka. If you make this into a cocktail, mix the vodka with the lime juice and passionfruit juice before adding the RoyalTEA.

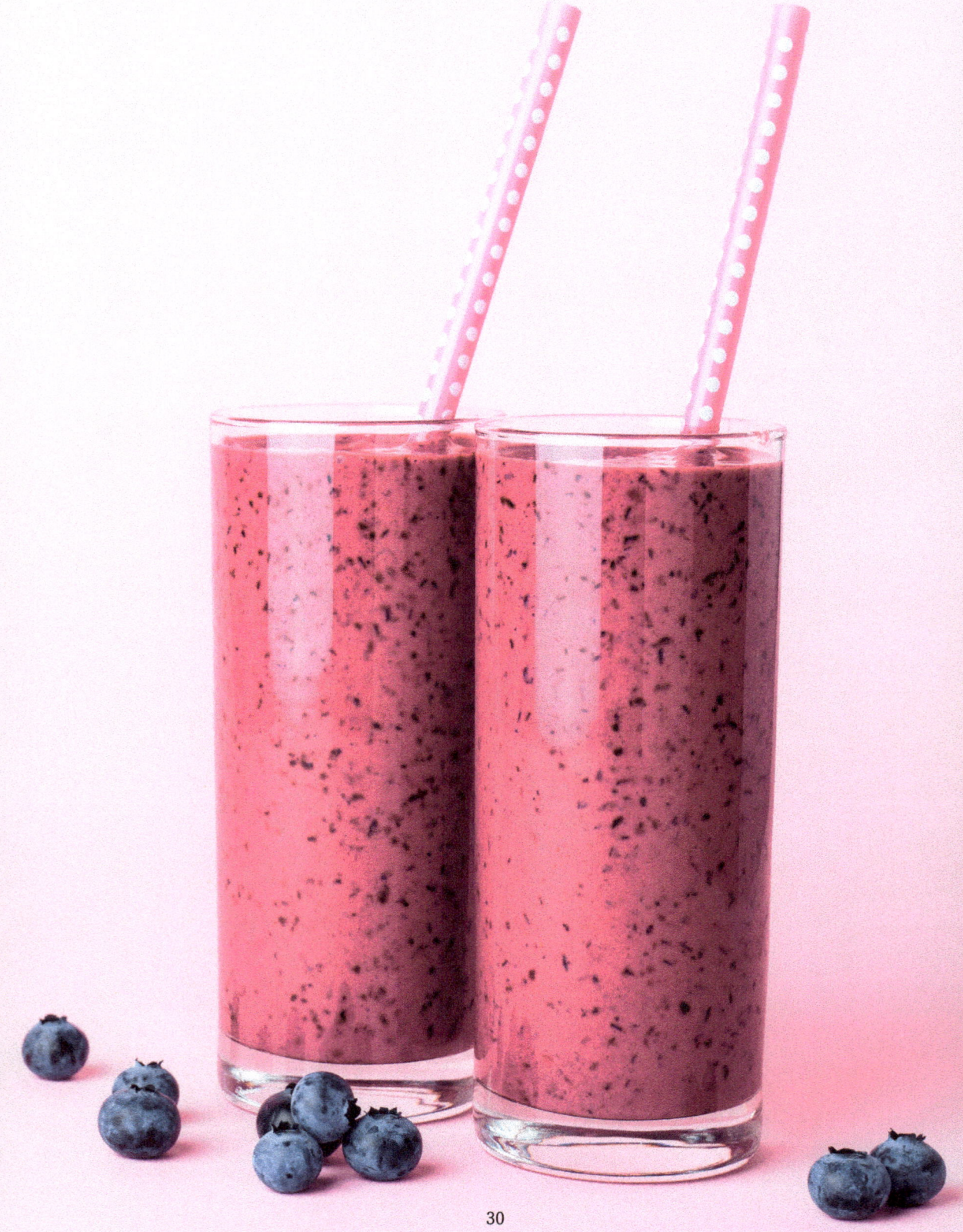

30

Royal Berry Blast

INGREDIENTS

Handful of Blueberries

Handful of Strawberries/Raspberries

Handful of Blackberries (optional)

1 ½ cup of Release Your RoyalTEA, brewed and sweetened to taste

INSTRUCTIONS

Combine ingredients in a blender.

Serve in your favorite glass or take on the go and enjoy!

Chapter 3

Release Your ImmuniTEA

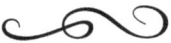

For years I suffered with chronic stress. It was during those times that I noticed I would get the worst colds that would linger for 2 weeks and sometimes develop into a sinus infection. I used my usual arsenal of natural remedies and even stepped it up a notch with IV vitamin infusions to no avail. Chronic stress compromises the immune system making you more susceptible to colds and other infections. Once I learned how to manage how I felt and responded to the stressful situations instead of the stressful situations controlling me, my stress began to dissipate. Then one day, the stressful situation was eliminated, and I started feeling a sense of FREEDOM.

I noticed that I wasn't getting colds anymore, but I still wanted to give my immune system a boost. I knew research showed that elderberry decreased the severity of symptoms and length of colds and flu, but what if I used it to help prevent that happening?

One of the best things you can do for your immune system is relax and rest. So, I blended elderberry with holy basil and other herbs and voila!

Release Your ImmuniTEA Ingredients:
- 🌿 Elderberry
- 🌿 Ginger Root
- 🌿 Holy Basil (aka Tulsi)
- 🌿 Hibiscus
- 🌿 Dried Blueberries

Release Your ImmuniTEA Benefits:
- Elderberries are a great source of potassium and vitamin.
- Ginger root is a natural anti-inflammatory
- Holy basil has antibacterial, antiviral, antifungal, and anti-inflammatory properties It protects the body and brain from the harmful effects of chronic stress, therefore it is classified as an adaptogen herb.
- Calming, positive effect on mood, natural anti-microbial enhances health and healing

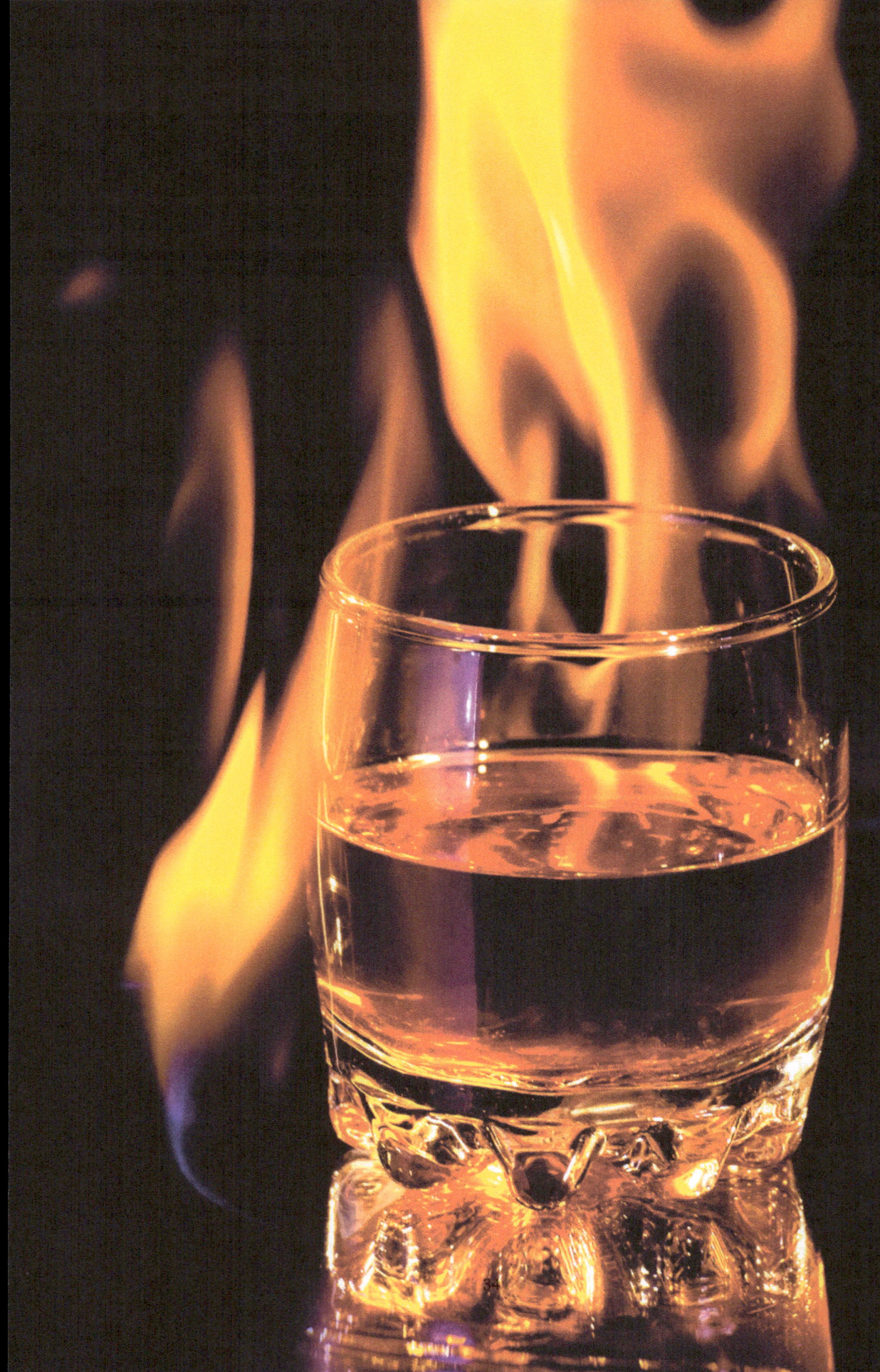

Bourbon Berry Bliss

INGREDIENTS

1 tbsp. Release Your ImmuniTEA

2 oz. Bourbon

1 oz. Amaretto

10 oz. Distilled or Spring Water

Honey to taste

INSTRUCTIONS

Bring water to a boil

Add 1 tablespoon of Release Your ImmuniTEA to pot or mug with hot water. (Can add tea to empty tea bags or loose in pan). Let steep for 7-10 minutes.

Using a strainer (or remove tea bags) strain the tea. Sweeten to taste. Not too much.

Add tea to two mugs dividing evenly.

Add 1 oz. of bourbon to each mug (or more if desired). Stir.

Top with a splash of Amaretto or to taste.

Enjoy warm and soothing.

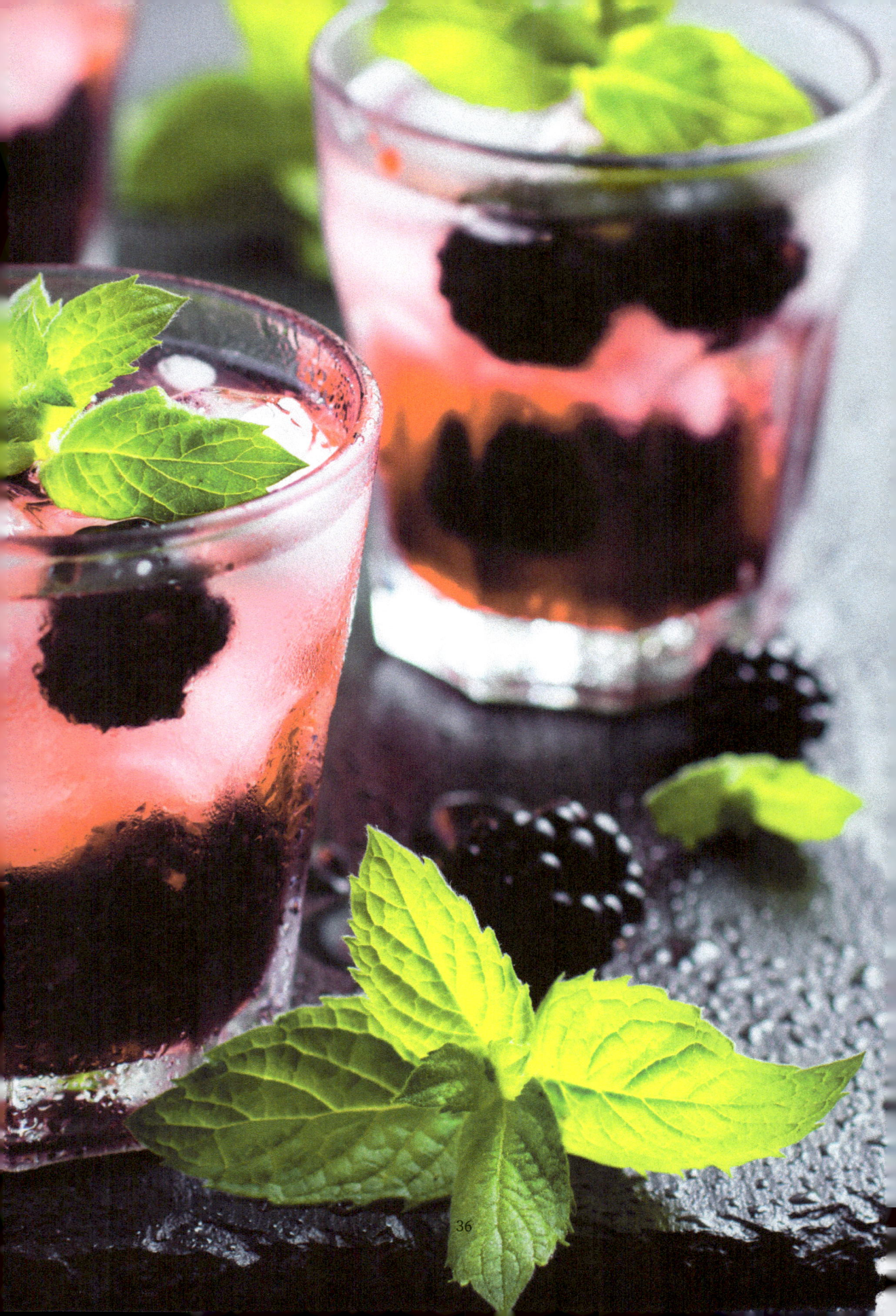

Release Your ImmuniTEA Tail

INGREDIENTS

¼ cup of Release Your ImmuniTEA simple syrup (you can add less or more depending on your preference)

1 cup of Caribbean rum (I prefer Babancourt Haitian rum)

Juice from 1 fresh squeezed lime

One handful of blackberries

3-5 mint sprigs

Tonic Water (optional)

INSTRUCTIONS

Muddle the blackberries

Combine Release Your ImmuniTEA simple syrup, rum blackberries, mint leaves, and lime juice in a cocktail shaker. Stir (or shake) and strain into a glass over ice.

Top off with a small amount of tonic water if tastes too sweet

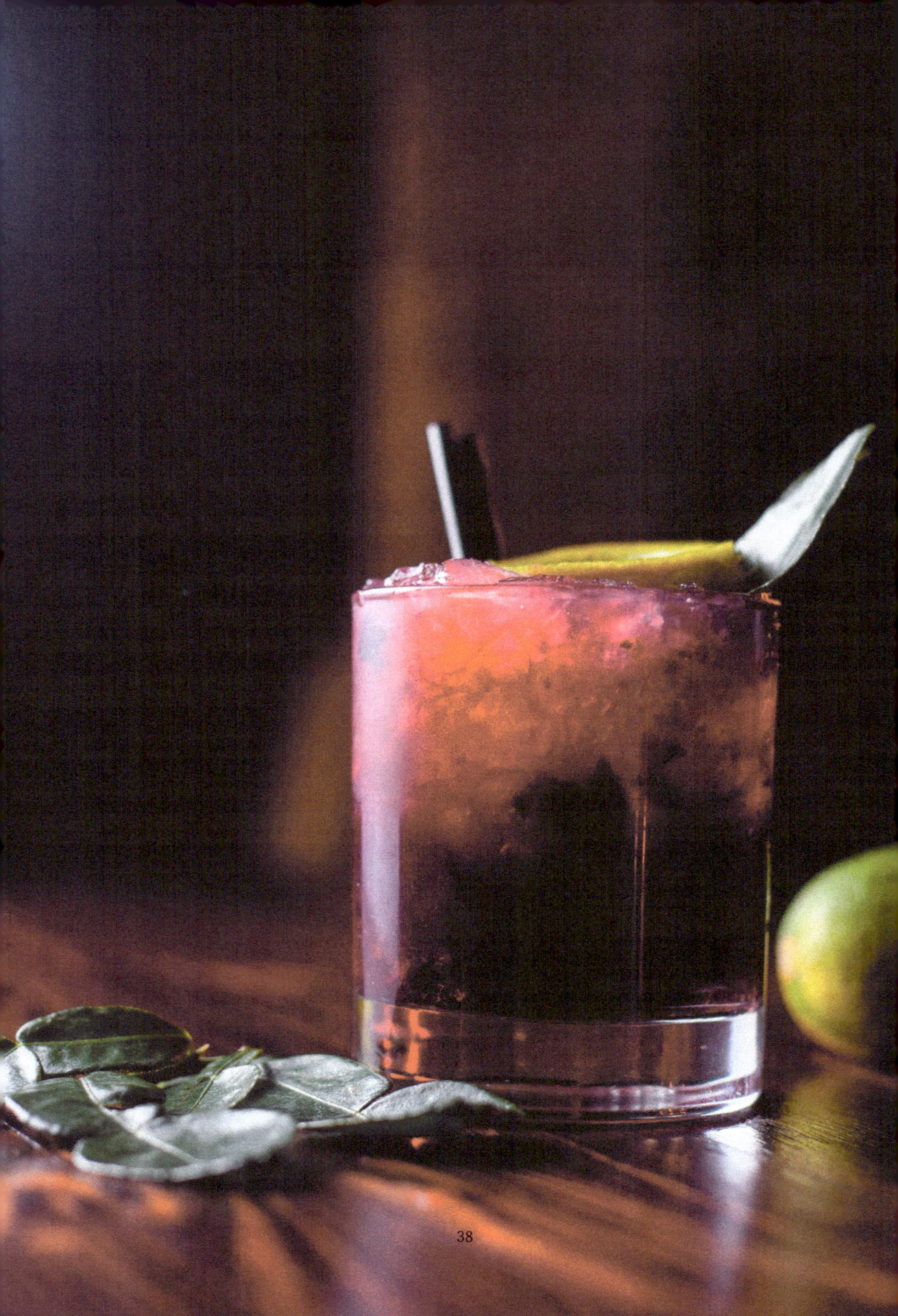

Immune Berry Spritzer

INGREDIENTS

1 handful of blueberries

1 handful of strawberries

1 handful of raspberries (optional)

honey or another sweetener such as agave

20 oz. of distilled or spring water

2 cups of Release Your ImmuniTEA Tea brewed, chilled

Club Soda/Pellegrino etc.

INSTRUCTIONS

Bring 20 ounces of water to a boil. Add 2 tablespoons of Release Your ImmuniTEA to pot (can add tea to empty tea bags or loose in pan). Let steep for 7-10 minutes.

Using a strainer (or remove tea bags) strain the tea. Sweeten to taste with honey/agave etc. Chill in the refrigerator for at least 1 hour.

In a glass add the berries. Using a wooden spoon or muddler, muddle the berries.

Add Release Your ImmuniTEA to glass about 2/3 full.

Pour back and forth between two glasses to adequately mix or use a cocktail shaker

Top with ice if desired.

Top off with a splash of club soda/ Pellegrino etc.

***OPTIONAL Make it a G&G (Good & Grown) spritzer by adding 2 ounces of your favorite gin (but don't sin)

Makes 2 servings

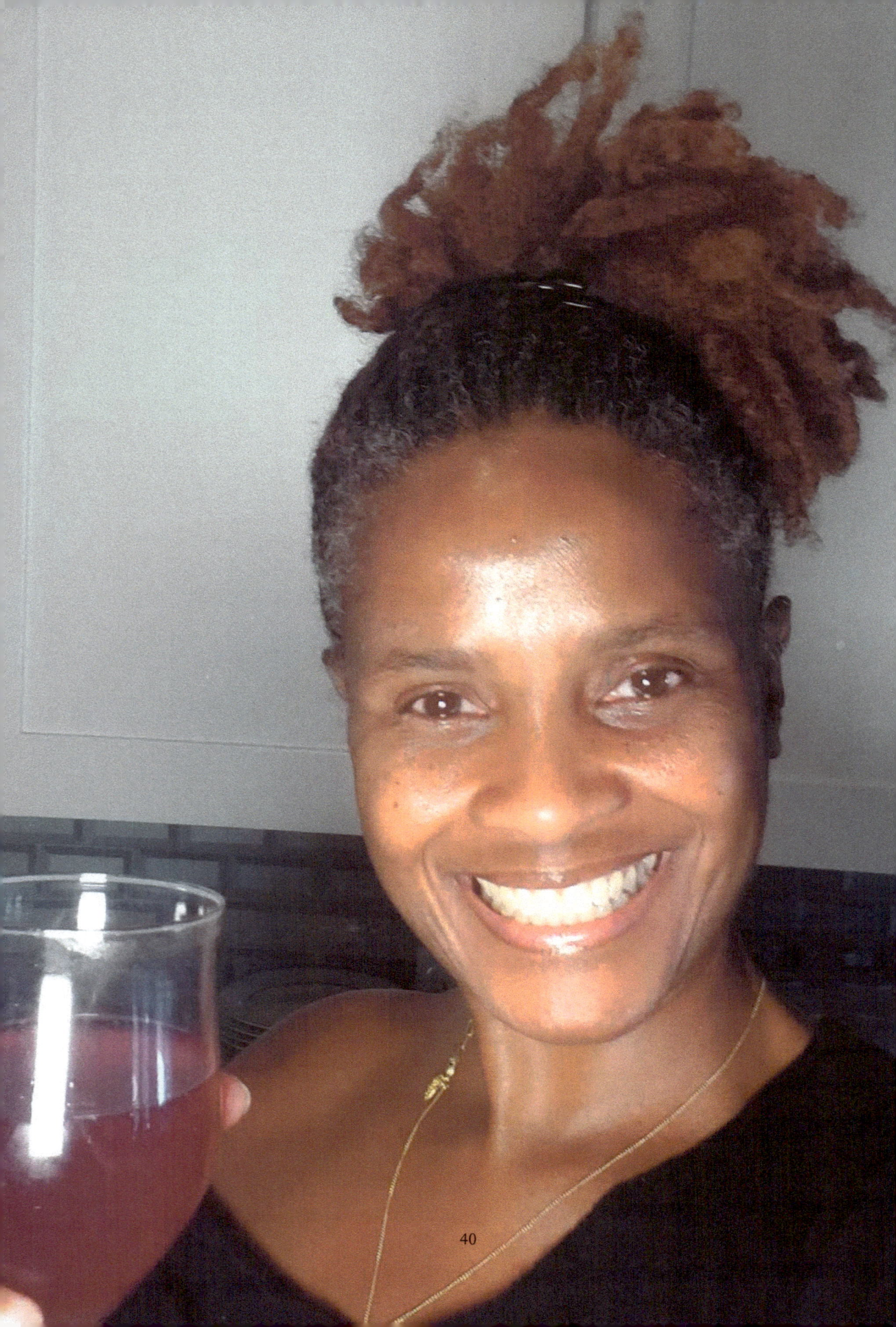

40

Berries & Bubbles

INGREDIENTS

2 tbsp. of Release Your ImmuniTEA

2 cups Distilled or Spring Water

4 oz. Blueberry Moscato

4 oz. Vodka

Rose Prosecco

INSTRUCTIONS

Bring 2 cups of water to a boil. Add 2 tablespoons of Release Your ImmuniTEA to pot (can add tea to empty tea bags or loose in pan). Let steep for 7-10 minutes.

Using a strainer (or remove tea bags) strain the tea. Sweeten to taste with honey/ agave etc. Not too sweet.

Chill in the refrigerator for at least 1 hour.

Mix Release Your ImmuniTEA, blueberry Moscato, and vodka in a pitcher. Stir

Pour into a chilled glass.

Top off with Rose Prosecco to desired amount.

CHEERS!

Makes 4 servings

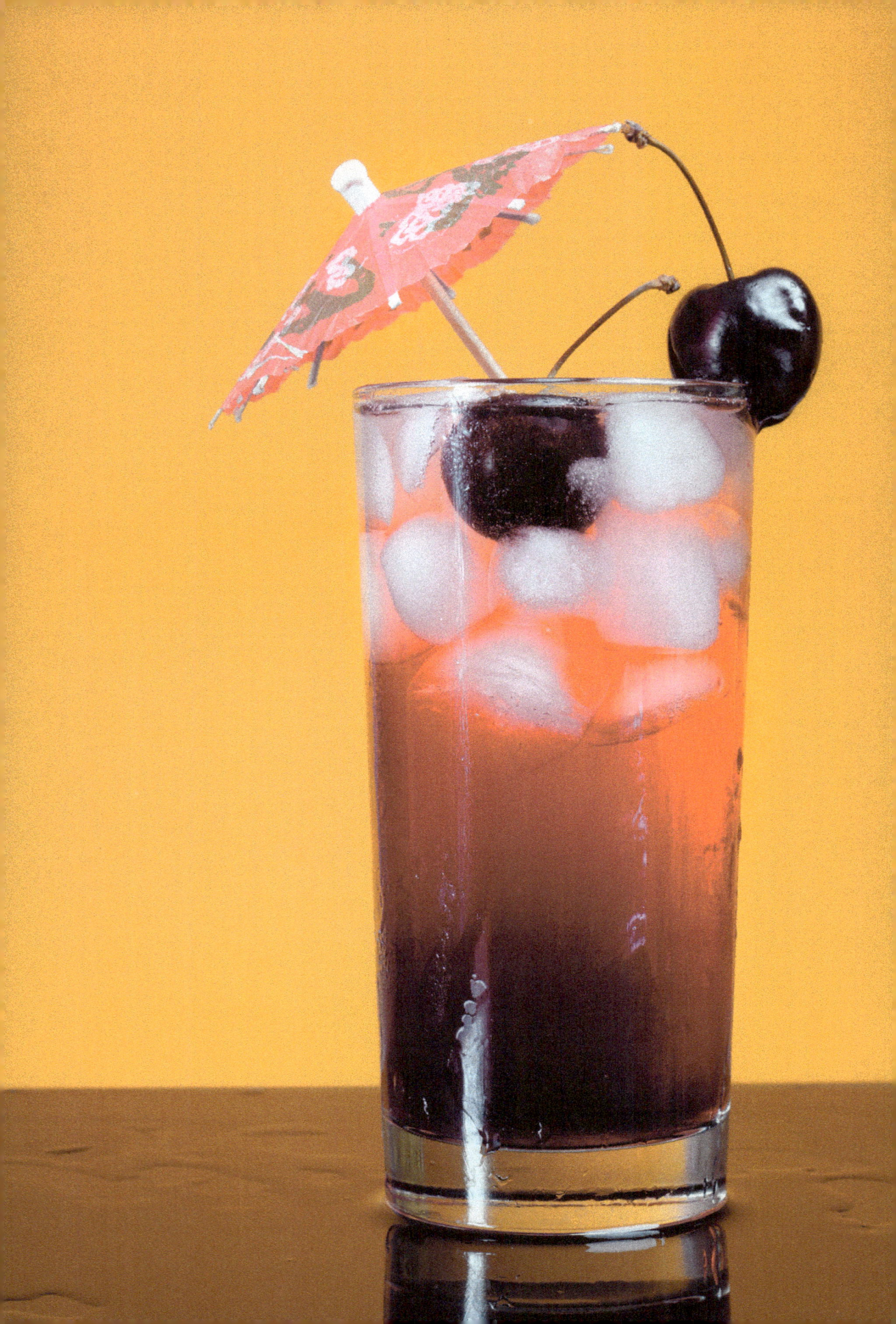

Berries & Cherries Spritzer

INGREDIENTS

2 tbsp. Release Your ImmuniTEA

5 fresh cherries, seed removed

Cherry or Pomegranate flavored sparkling water

Rose' (optional)

INSTRUCTIONS

Bring 2 cups of water to a boil. Add 2 tablespoons of Release Your ImmuniTEA to pot (can add tea to empty tea bags or loose in pan). Let steep for 7-10 minutes.

Using a strainer (or remove tea bags) strain the tea. Sweeten to taste with honey/agave etc. Chill in the refrigerator for at least 1 hour or you will need ice.

In a beverage shaker, add sliced cherries and a small amount of brewed Release Your ImmuniTEA. Muddle the fruit with a muddler or wooden spoon.

Once cherries are thoroughly muddled, add remaining Release Your ImmuniTEA. Shake, strain, and pour into two glasses.

Top with sparkling water and enjoy!

OPTIONS

* You can blend the cherries with Release Your ImmuniTEA instead of muddling if you want a stronger flavor

** You can add your favorite rose' to this or substitute it for the sparkling water.

Chapter 4

Release & Relieve

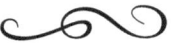

I often tell people I'm a root worker. I work with turmeric root, ginger root, dandelion root, and getting to the root of a matter. The tea blend Release & Relieve is all about roots. It was born out of a need to relieve the root cause of my pain and discomfort, which was inflammation from a car accident. My neck, shoulders, mid and lower back were as tight as a drum from the accident where I couldn't stand up straight. I was slowly walking around bent over like a 99-year-old woman when I was only 44. That wasn't going to work. I started juicing fresh ginger root, turmeric root, lemon juice, cinnamon, greens, and coconut oil when I was unable to take the muscle relaxants because they made me feel too loopy. It worked. Between my miracle root juice and the infrared sauna, I was starting to move more like myself. Once I returned to work, I had to figure out an easier way to transport this miracle root juice, so I did it in dry form to create this tea blend. I named it Release & Relieve because it helped me release inflammation and tight muscles and relieved my pain and discomfort.

Release & Relieve Ingredients:
- ❋ Turmeric Root
- ❋ Ginger Root
- ❋ Dried Lemon Slices
- ❋ Cinnamon
- ❋ Black Pepper

Release & Relieve Benefits:
- We already know about the powerful anti-inflammatory properties of turmeric root. Studies have shown its benefit with osteoarthritis. But turmeric root also helps brain function by increasing the production of brain-derived neurotrophic factor (BDNF). BDNF plays a role in improving memory, learning, and attention. Turmeric is an integral part of your healing and cleansing journey. It protects the liver from damage, while supporting the regeneration of liver cells.
- Ginger root is a natural anti-inflammatory. Studies show that it can reduce pain and discomfort from osteoarthritis, especially in the knees. Ginger

root has other health benefits such as helping to lower blood sugar and cholesterol levels. If experiencing nausea or indigestion, ginger can help alleviate these symptoms

- Lemon is a go to food when treating anemia. While there is a small amount of iron in lemons, consuming lemons with other plant-based foods rich in iron helps the body absorb the iron better.
- Soothing, improve digestive health, enhance health and wellness.

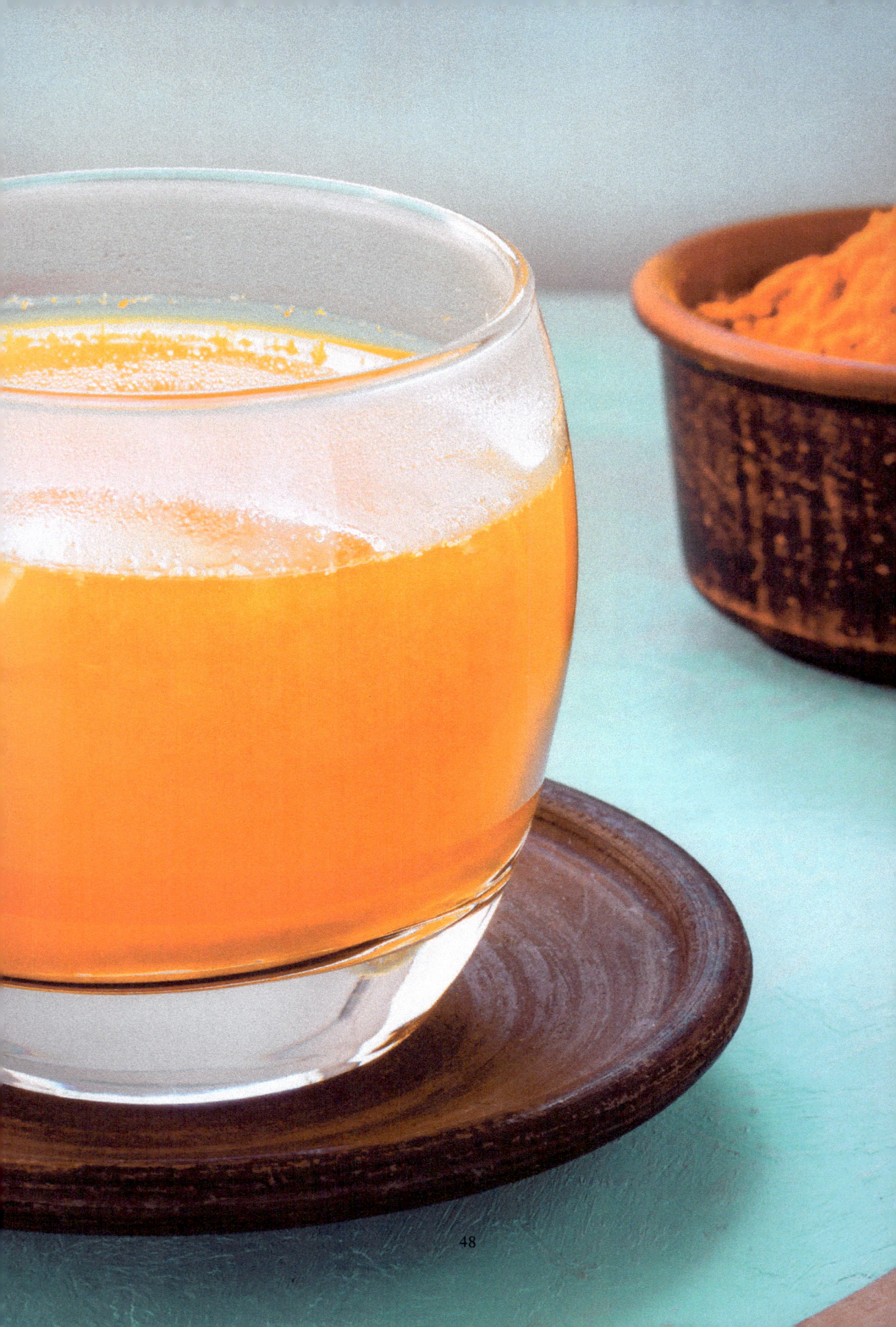

Rum Ease

INGREDIENTS

1 tbsp. Release & Relieve

10oz. Distilled or Spring Water

Cayenne Pepper

Honey

Malibu Rum

INSTRUCTIONS

Bring 10 ounces of hot water to a boil. Add 1 tbsp of Release & Relieve tea. Allow to steep for 5-7 minutes

Add honey to taste

Add a dash of cayenne pepper

Add 1 ounce of Malibu rum

Sit back sip and allow the flavors to soothe your body, mind, and soul.

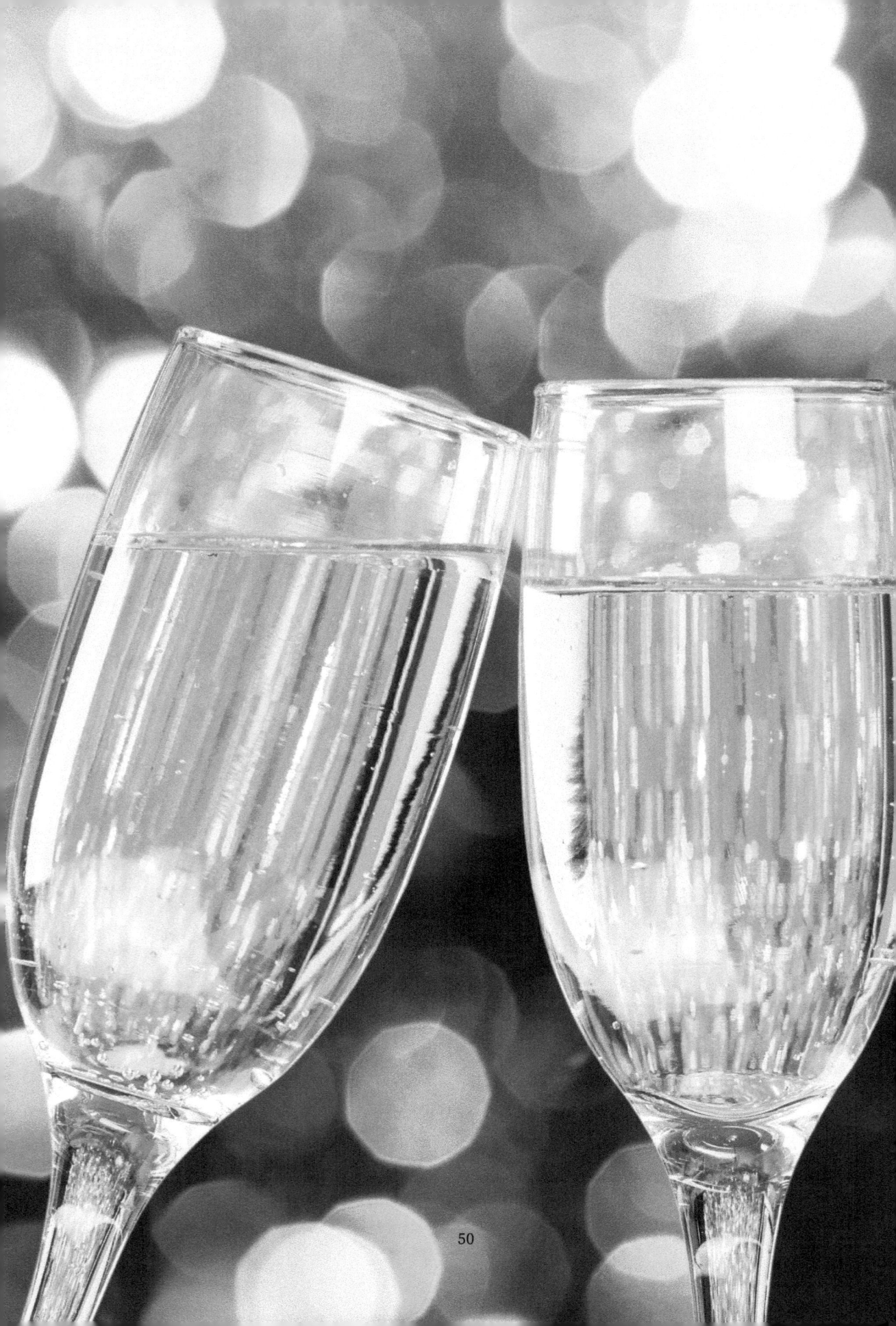

Release Relieve & Sparkle

INGREDIENTS

¼ cup Release & Relieve simple syrup

½ cup fresh squeezed orange juice, chilled

1 bottle Champagne, chilled (can substitute Prosecco or any sparkling wine)

Garnish (optional):

Orange slices

Cinnamon sticks

Edible "glitter"

INSTRUCTIONS

Run an orange slice around the rim of each champagne flute or any stemmed glass. Place the edible "glitter" into a small plate or dish. Dip and turn the rims of each glass into the sugar. Set aside.

Add about 2 tablespoons each of the orange juice and simple syrup into each glass. Top off each glass with champagne. Garnish with an orange slice or cinnamon stick.

*NOTE For a mocktail, replace the champagne with sparkling white grape, pear, or apple juice.

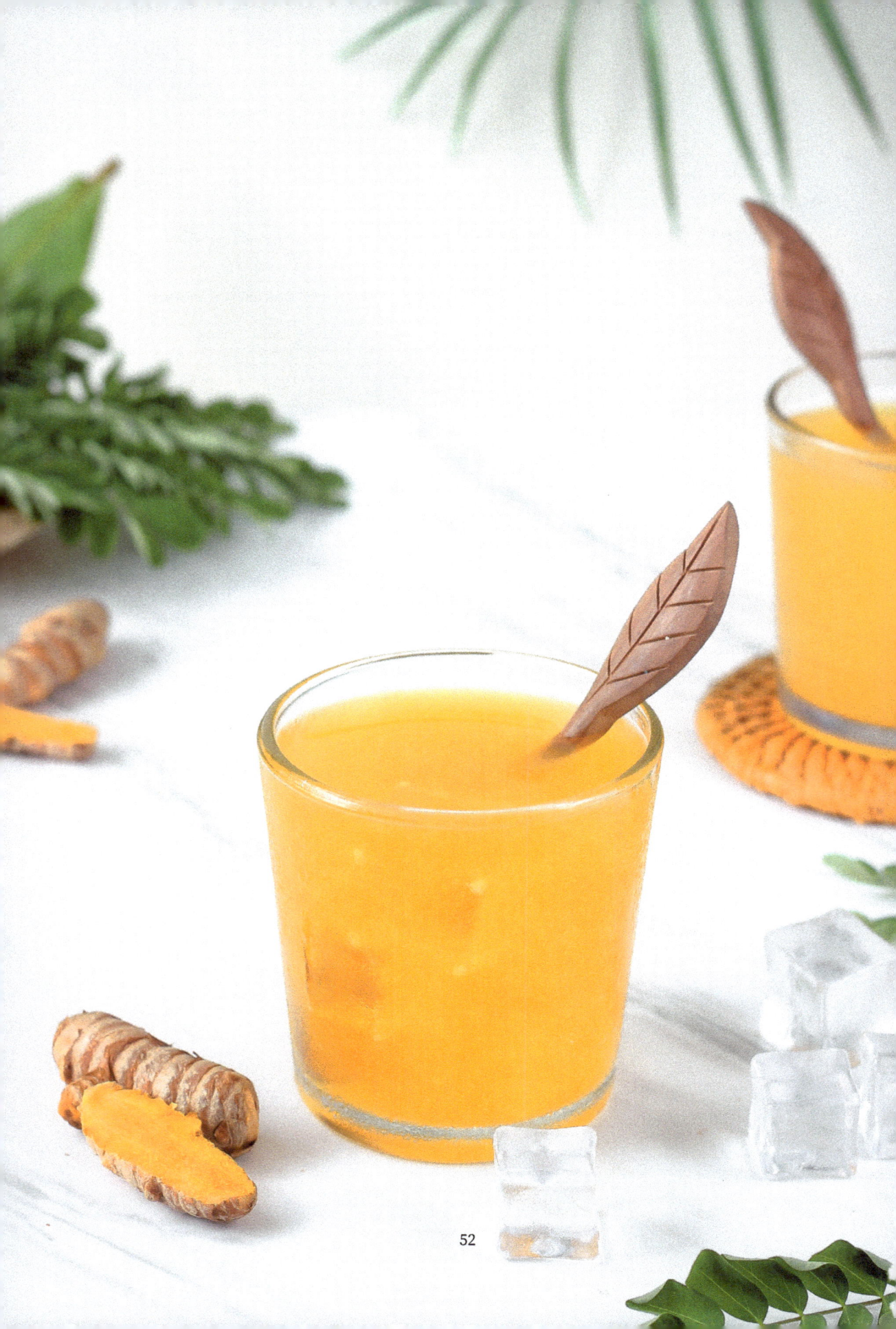

RootTEAni

INGREDIENTS

6 tbsp of Release & Relieve Tea

6 cups of water

3 cups ice cubes

25 oz. of Vodka

2 cups of Ginger Beer

Honey to taste

INSTRUCTIONS

Bring 6 cups of water to a boil. Once has reached the boiling point. Turn off the heat and add tea.

Let steep for 10 minutes.

Add honey and stir if desire a sweeter taste

Place in refrigerator to cool

Fill a large glass pitcher or punch bowl about ½ way with ice cubes. Pitcher should hold about two gallons.

Pour in the cooled tea then add the vodka and ginger beer.

Stir it well with a long spoon then set it out to serve in 4-ounce glasses. Guests can add ice to their cup, then serve the punch from the pitcher.

Garnish with mint and lime

Makes 14 servings

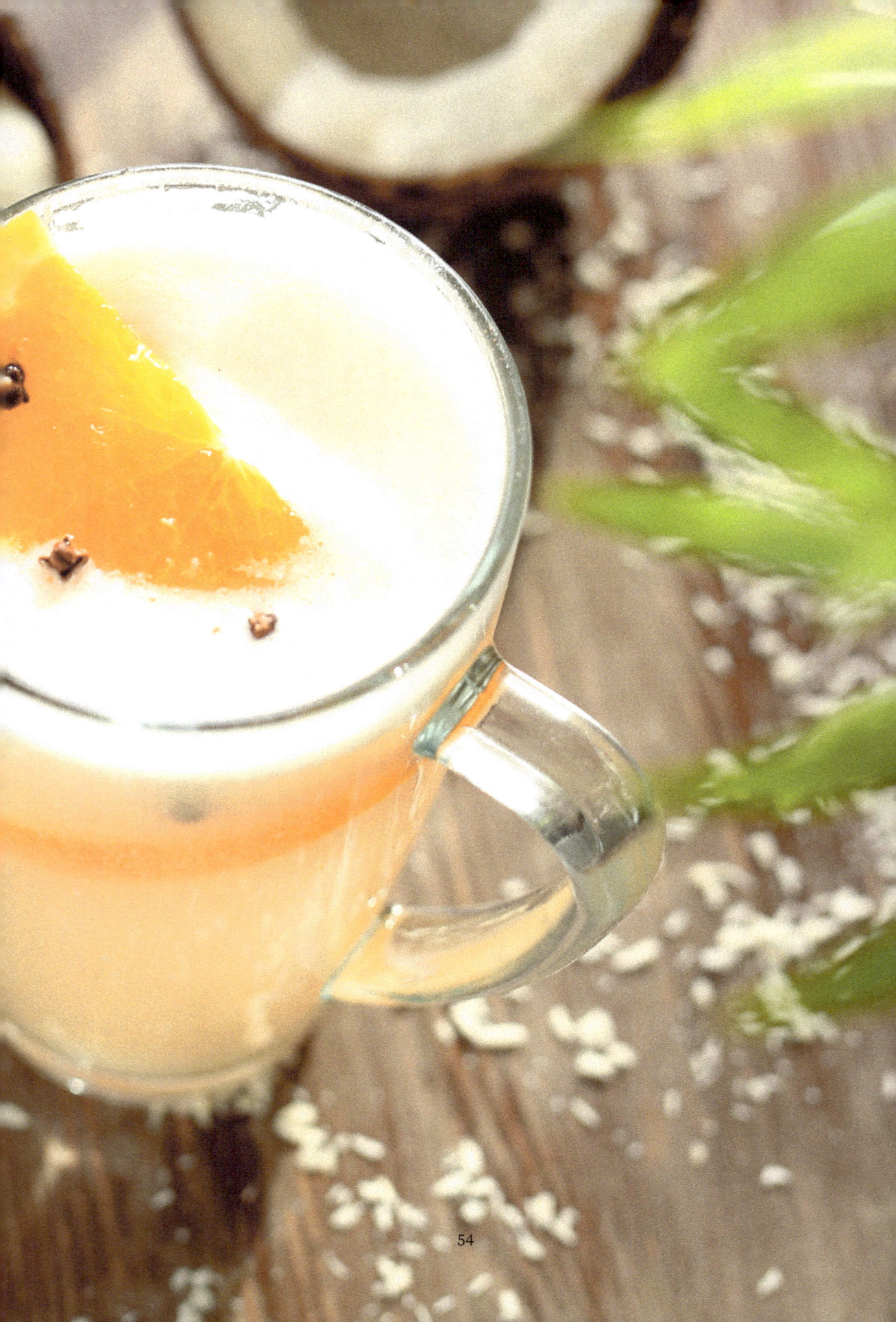

Coco Relief Smoothie

INGREDIENTS

2 tbsp. Release & Relieve simple syrup

1 cup Vitacoco Coconut water

½ Orange

Handful of spinach or kale

INSTRUCTIONS

Add ½ an orange, coconut water, 1 tablespoon of Release & Relieve simple syrup, and spinach to blender.

Blend until thoroughly mixed.

Pour into a nice glass and enjoy!

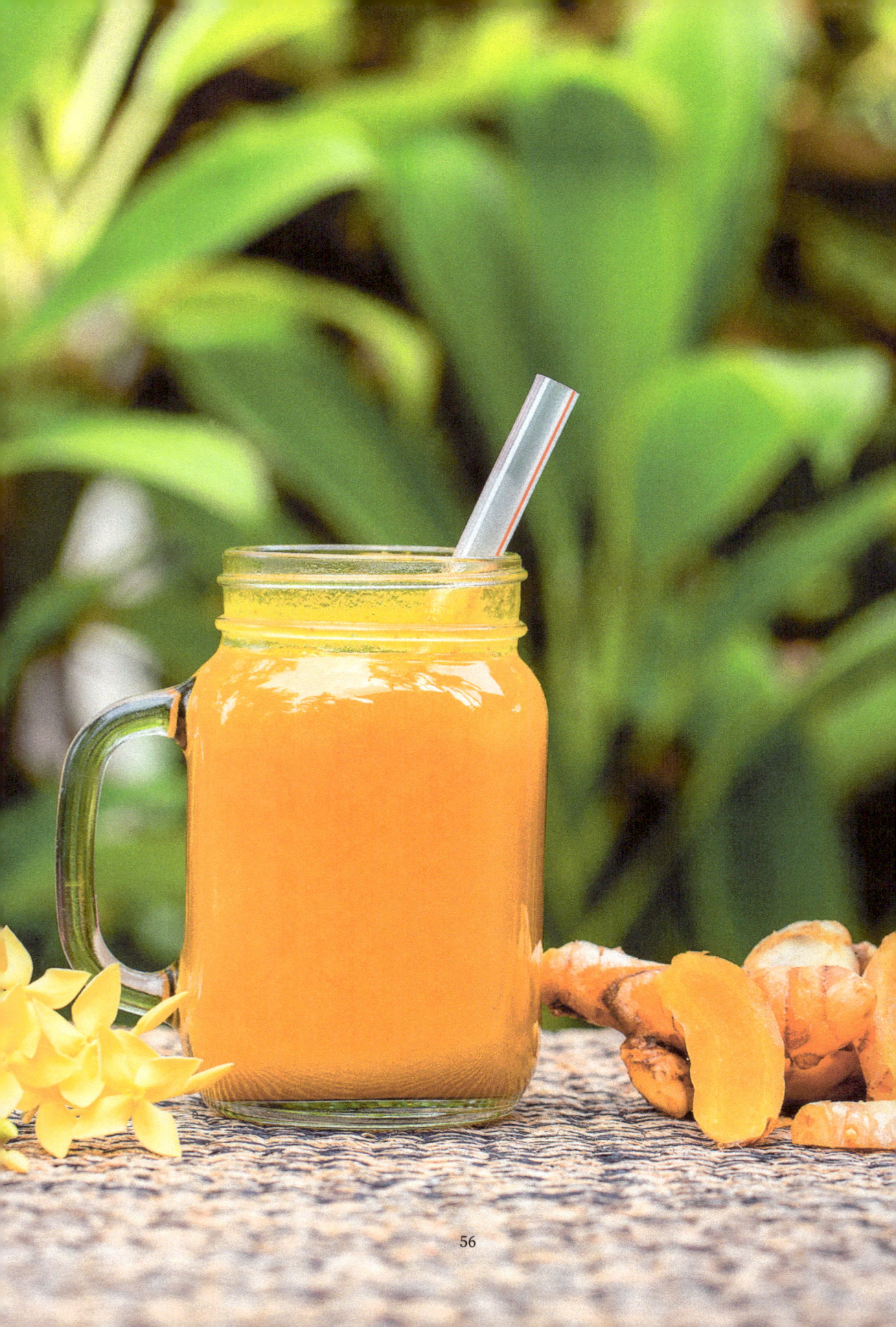

Release & Relieve Turmeric Smoothie

INGREDIENTS

1 ¼ cup Distilled or Spring Water

1 tbsp Release & Relieve tea

1 handful of leafy greens (spinach, kale etc.)

1 kiwi

½ mango

Honey

INSTRUCTIONS

Boil water. Once boiled, add Release & Relieve tea.

Steep and let cool. Once cooled, strain tea and set aside to cool completely.

*NOTE this can be made ahead of time to cool completely and chill.

Place all ingredients in a high-powered blender and blend thoroughly.

*Optional add honey or another sweetener to taste

Serve and enjoy!

Chapter 5

Release & Purify Green Tea

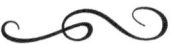

Green tea is gaining momentum in the Western world, after being a staple in Asian countries for centuries. Green tea became very important to me when my doctor referred me to a breast specialist after a mammogram. My mammogram was normal, but due to a very strong family history of breast cancer (my mother and my aunt), she thought it best to be thorough. I saw a breast specialist and a geneticist. I declined the test for BRCA, the genetic marker for breast cancer. Instead, I decided to take my health destiny into my own hands by being intentional about everything I consumed physically through food, emotionally through relationships and minimizing my stress as much as possible. That's when I started drinking green tea 2-3 times per day. It was not a pleasant experience; it tasted like grass (well the smell of grass, I've never actually tasted it). Being the alchemist and healing helper that I am, I knew I could create something that was helpful and healthful while being pleasant to consume. I combined the two top-quality green tea varieties with orange peel and mango powder to smooth out the taste. The flavor alone or in combination with fruits as a smoothie or spirits as a cocktail is DIVINELY delicious.

Release & Purify Green Tea Ingredients:

- ❦ Sencha Green Tea
- ❦ Matcha Green Tea
- ❦ Moringa Leaves
- ❦ Yarrow Flowers
- ❦ Orange Peel
- ❦ Mango Powder

Release & Purify Green Tea Benefits:

- There are over 150 varieties of green tea. Release & Purify Green tea is made with two of the top-quality types, sencha and matcha. It's best to drink green tea as opposed to taking green tea supplements. Green tea supports cleansing and a detoxification program by protecting the liver from damage caused by toxic substances such as alcohol or Tylenol. Green tea also suppresses the appetite and helps burn fat cells in combination with exercise.

- One of the active ingredients in green tea called L-Theanine, suppresses the stress response supporting calmer feelings while also increasing focus and concentration.

- Yarrow flowers help alleviate digestive symptoms such as bloating, diarrhea, constipation, and stomach pain. *** Caution: people allergic to ragweed should avoid yarrow.

- Moringa is considered the "king of herbs". It is extremely nutritious containing 25 times more iron than spinach, 17 times more calcium than milk, and 4 times more protein than eggs. Moringa has a lowering effect on blood sugar and cholesterol

- Energizing improves focus and concentration, recharges health and wellness.

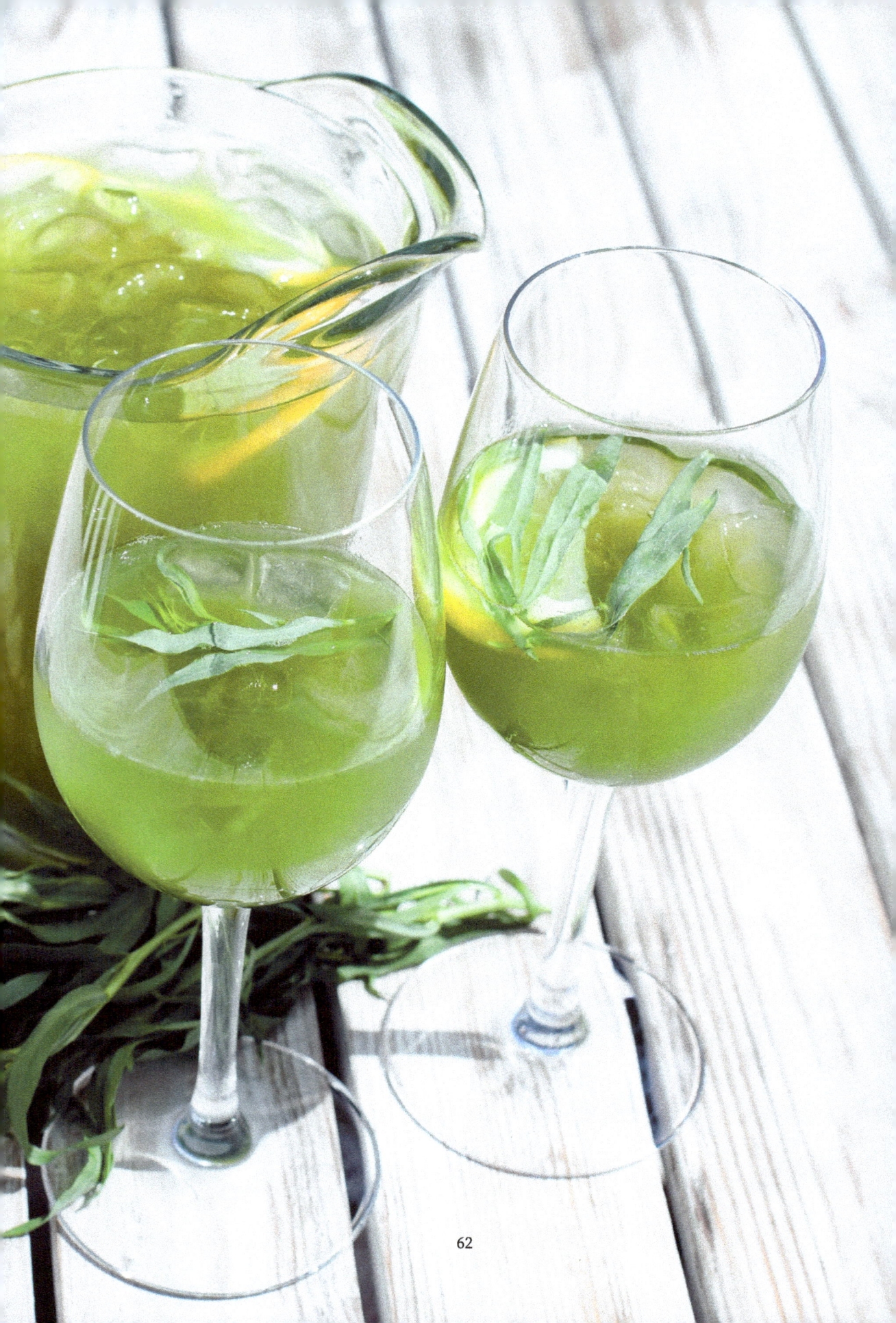

PuriTEA Green Lemonade

INGREDIENTS

1 Tbsp. Release & Purify Green Tea

2 cups of Fresh water (spring or distilled)

Juice of 3 lemons

½ cup of Cilantro

4 tbsp. Honey

INSTRUCTIONS

Bring water to 175 degrees.

Add Release & Purify Green tea to a tea bag. Add tea bag to water and allow to steep for 5 minutes. Remove tea and allow to cool completely.

Once cooled, add 1 cup to a blender. Add cilantro and blend.

Strain leaves if desired.

Add honey to lemon juice in a separate mixing glass. Mix well.

Add tea with cilantro to lemon honey mixture. Stir well.

Divide between 2 glasses and enjoy.

OPTIONS

- This recipe may be substituted with basil leaves.
- You can add your favorite spirit such as vodka or gin to make the G & G and version.
- Use as much honey as desired for your taste

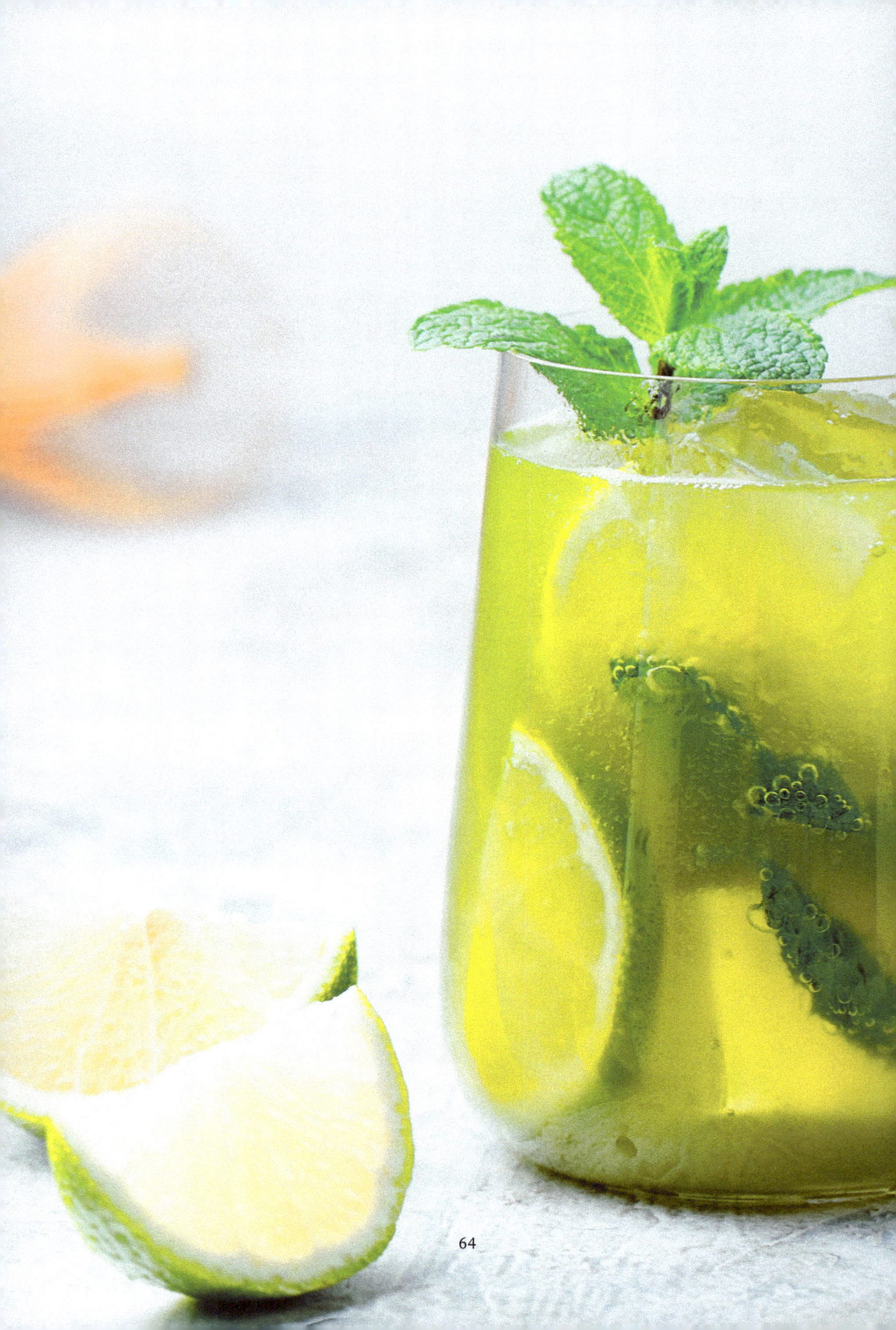

Fancy FREETEAni

INGREDIENTS

1 tbsp Release & Purify Green Tea

2 cups Distilled or Spring Water

Tito's vodka

Lime

INSTRUCTIONS

Heat 16 ounces of water to 150 – 180 degrees. Add 1 tablespoon of Release & Purify Green tea to a tea bag. Add tea bag to water and allow to steep for 5 minutes. Remove tea and allow to cool completely.

Chill in the refrigerator for at least 1 hour.

Once the tea has chilled, in a fresh glass, add Tito's and 1 cup of Release & Purify Green tea.

Cut a lime wedge and squeeze fresh juice.

CHEERS!

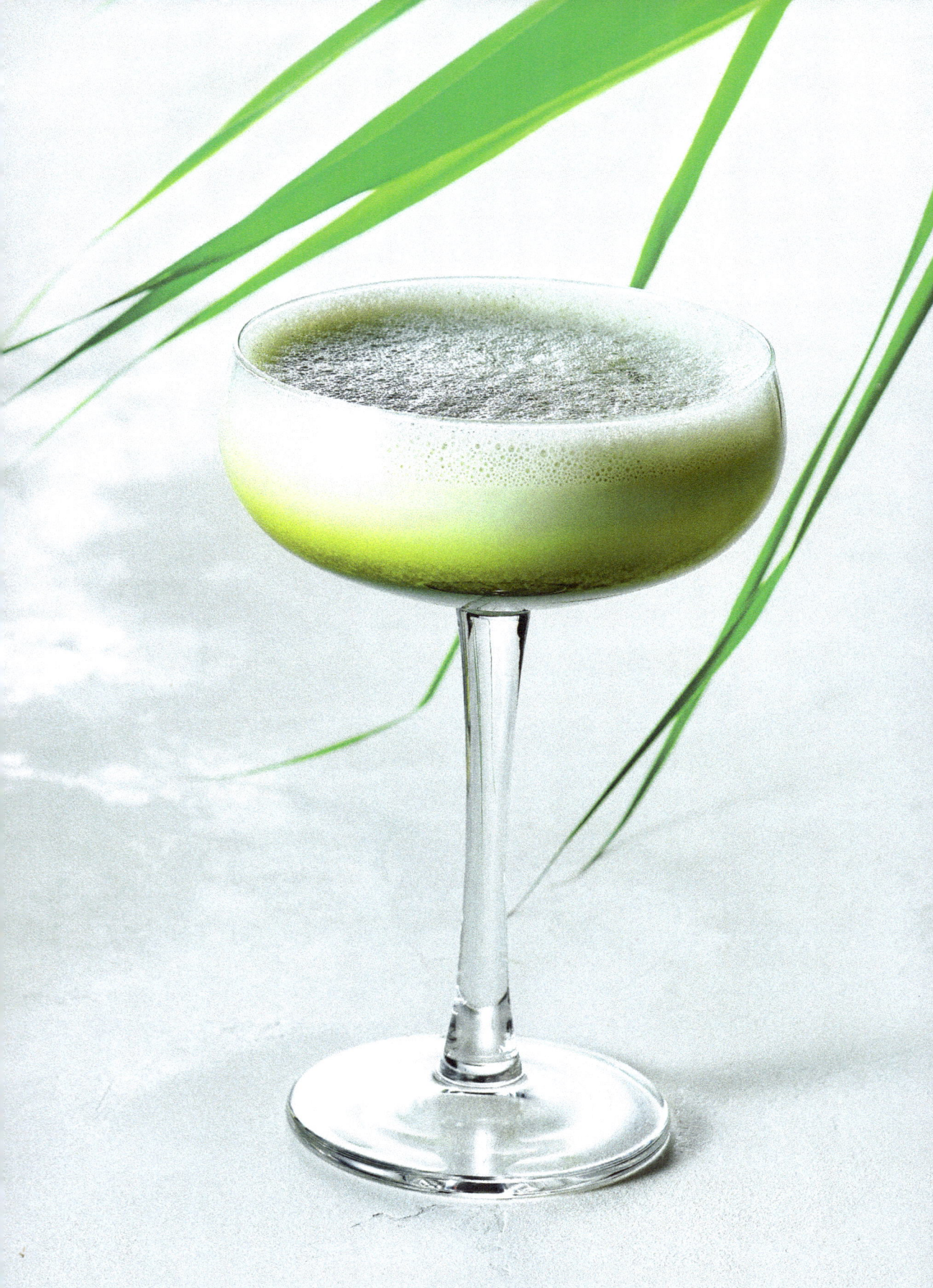

Pineapple Puritini

INGREDIENTS

¾ cup of Release & Purify Green tea, brewed and chilled

2 ounces vodka

5 chunks of fresh pineapple

Juice of ¼ of an orange

Juice of ½ of a lime

INSTRUCTIONS

Add vodka and pineapple to a cocktail shaker and muddle. Add crushed ice, then all remaining ingredients. Shake to combine and pour into a martini glass.

CHEERS!

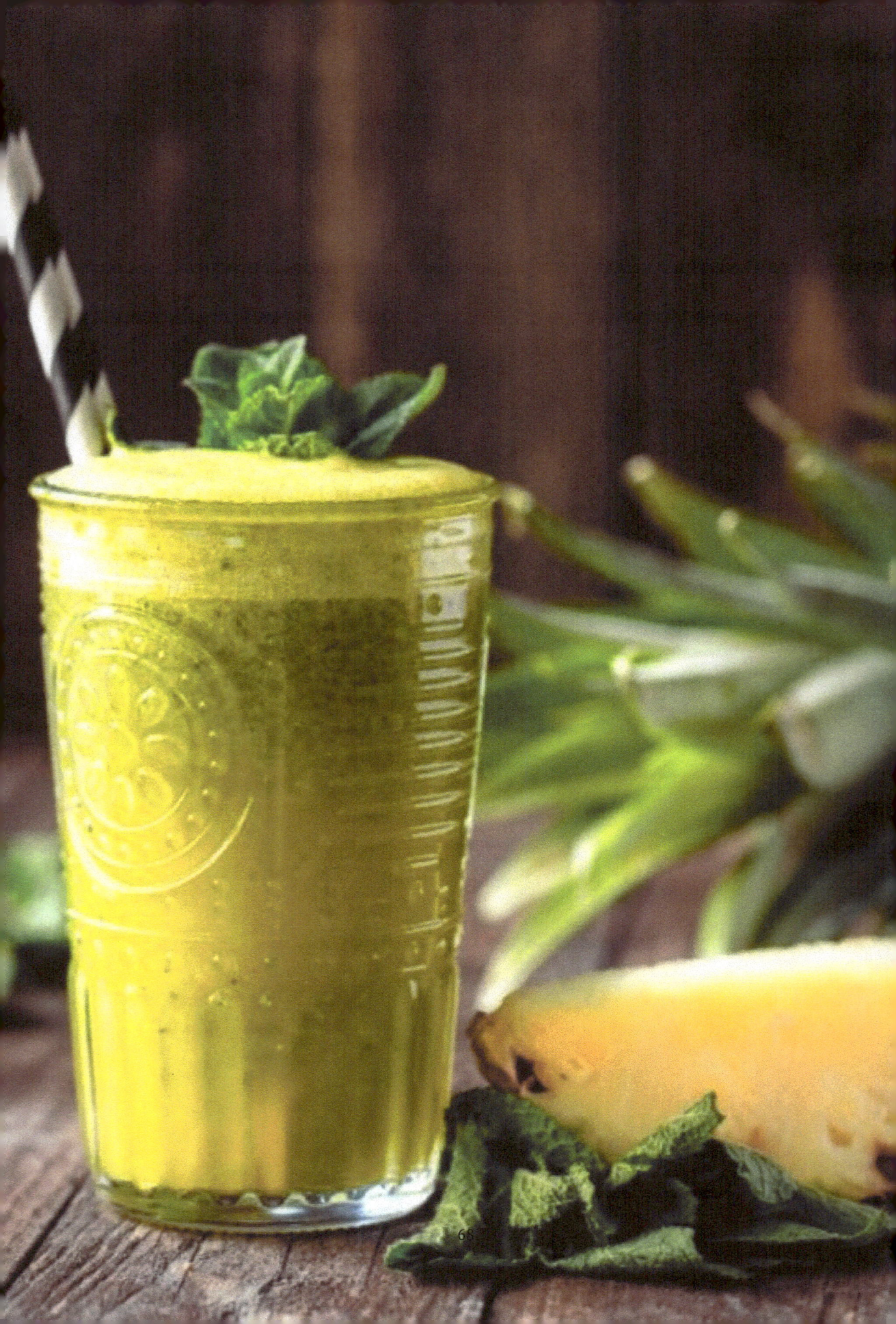

Purify & Pineapple Smoothie

INGREDIENTS

Release & Purify Green Tea (brewed & chilled)

½ - ¾ cup of Pineapple Chunks

1 Kiwi, peeled

Juice of 1 Lemon

2 Kale Leaves

Distilled Water

INSTRUCTIONS

Heat water to no hotter than 170 degrees. Add ½ tablespoon of Release & Purify Green Tea to a tea bag. Add tea bag to water and allow to steep for 5 minutes. Remove tea and allow to cool completely.

Add all ingredients to include chilled Release & Purify Green Tea to a blender

Blend until smooth

Add more tea or water, if necessary, to desired consistency

Optional add honey to taste

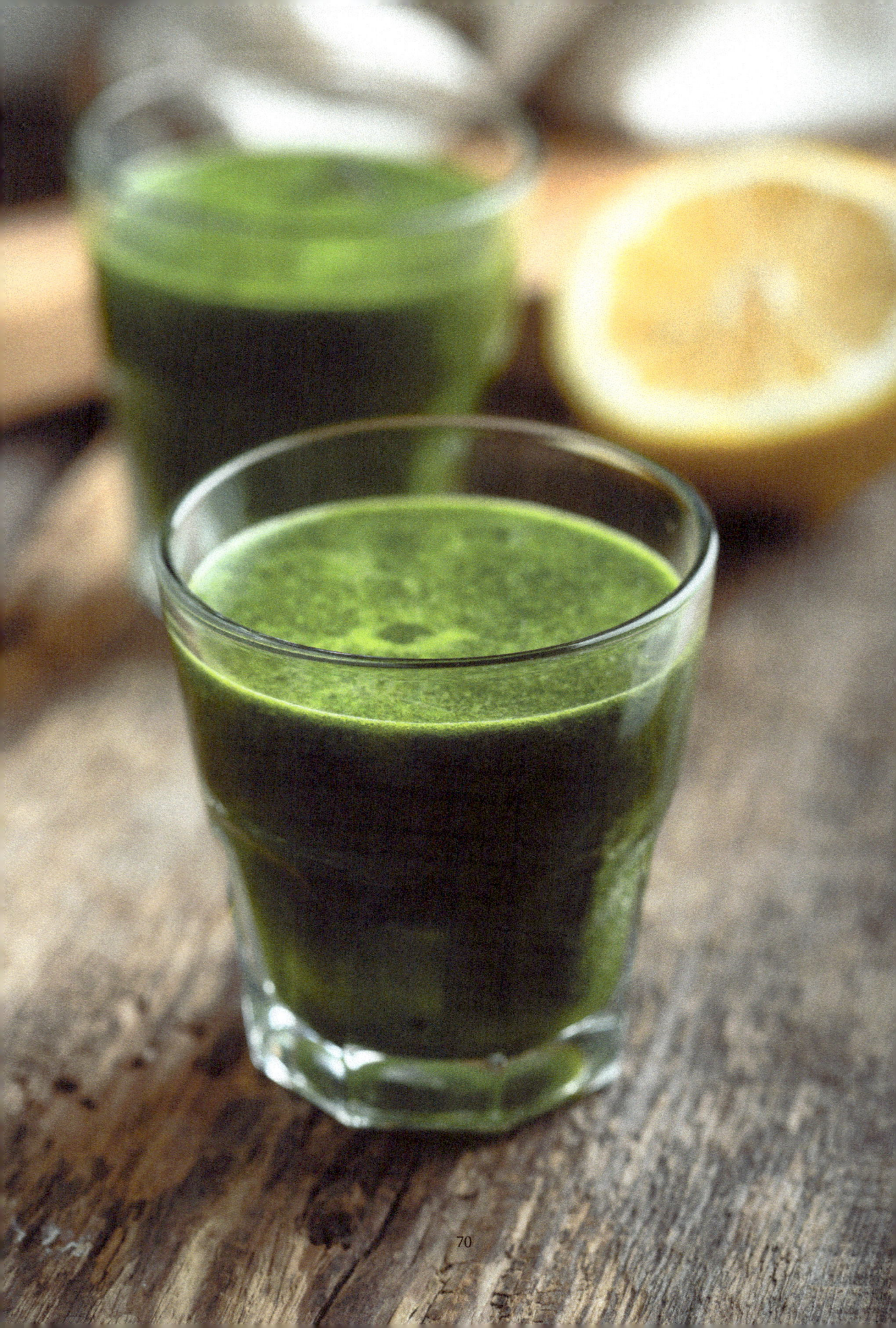

Purify Green Dream Juice

INGREDIENTS

Release & Purify Green Tea (brewed and chilled)

1 stalk of Celery

2-3 leaves of Lacinato Kale

Juice of ½ lemon

Honey or agave

Distilled water

INSTRUCTIONS

Heat 10 ounces of water to 150 – 180 degrees. Add ½ tablespoon of Release & Purify Green Tea to a tea bag. Add tea bag to water and allow to steep for 5 minutes. Remove tea and allow to cool completely.

Chill in refrigerator for 45 minutes – 1 hour.

Add ½ of the chilled tea to a blender. Add 1 stalk of celery and kale leaves cleaned and cut up to easily blend. Blend. Strain through a sifter. Add honey to taste and lemon juice. Stir and ENJOY!

Chapter 6

Release Rise & Shine

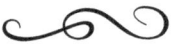

Years ago, I saw the power of fresh whole foods in action. My mother was diagnosed with breast cancer. She waited to seek treatment until the tumor had grown so large, it started eroding through her skin. There was blood, pus, and an odor that smelled like dying flesh. Once she finally sought treatment, it entailed MANY weeks of chemo, a mastectomy, and radiation. It was in remission for 3 ½ years. But once it returned, it came back with a vengeance! It metastasized to her brain. Another round of radiation left her exhausted and depleted. I asked her what she wanted to do. She responded, "I've done everything the doctors have told me to do. I want to try something natural this time."

In walks Mr. Hank Jones & Mrs. Yemi Bates-Jones. I met them through a gentleman I met on a 14-day trip to Egypt. He told me he would introduce me to his teachers who may be able to help my mother. After speaking to them, they agreed they could help her on her journey which would require us to come to Cottonwood, Alabama. I flew from Philadelphia where I was living at the time to Indianapolis to pick up my mother. When I arrived at the house, it looked like a nursing home. There was a wheelchair, walker, canes, and items to assist bathing. She couldn't drive, dress herself, and she could not conceptualize front from back with her shirts and pants. I was shocked and scared because she never revealed how bad she was feeling even though we talked at least once per day.

Once we arrived in Cottonwood, they immediately began feeding us whole, fresh foods, mostly raw. We consumed a lot of juices and different types of herbal teas and tinctures. Week after week, I saw improvements with my mother. After 4 weeks, my mother was showering by herself, shopping, and she even went back to work. I was amazed! I had the honor of watching her miraculous transformation.

Since I was consuming most of the same things she was, I experienced a transformation as well. I felt a lift and a rise in my body, soul, and mind! I knew that I would never go back to living the way I was prior to this encounter in Cottonwood, Alabama at the Purification Garden. That is the inspiration for Release Rise & Shine tea. It started as a fresh juice with hand-squeezed lemon, orange, grapefruit, and ginger root. I made this in dry form with the substitution of dandelion root for grapefruit juice.

This tea is great for the digestive system and immune health.

Release Rise & Shine Tea Ingredients:
- ❧ Dried Orange Slices
- ❧ Orange Peel
- ❧ Lemon Peel
- ❧ Ginger Root
- ❧ Dandelion Root

Release Rise & Shine Tea Benefits:

- Orange peel provides three times the amount of Vitamin C compared to the inner pulp. Diets high in Vitamin C improve heart health and mitigate spikes in the stress hormone cortisol when events trigger the stress response.

- Lemon peel has anti-microbial properties that can contribute to better oral health by fighting common bacteria that cause oral disease. Due to its high Vitamin C and flavonoid content, lemon peel can boost the immune system and decrease the length and severity of symptoms of the common cold.

- Ginger root is a natural anti-inflammatory. Studies show that it can reduce pain and discomfort from osteoarthritis, especially in the knees. Ginger root has other health benefits such as helping to lower blood sugars and cholesterol levels. If experiencing nausea or indigestion, ginger can help alleviate these symptoms

- Dandelion root has a mild laxative effect and is used to improve digestion and relieves gas and constipation. It also improves the function of the liver and gall bladder.

- Energizing, improve digestive health, enhance health and wellness.

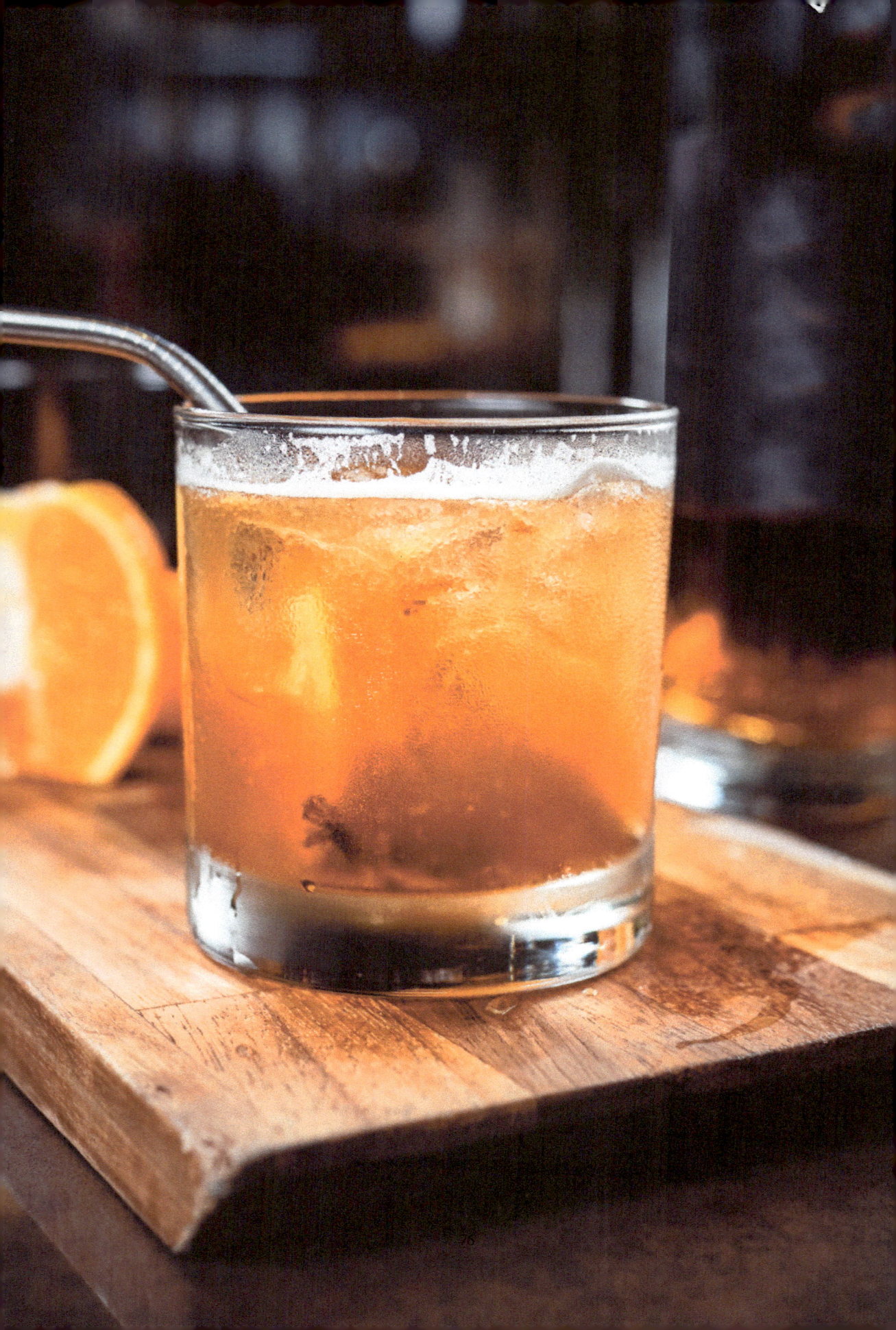

Rise & Shine Toddy

INGREDIENTS

4 tbsp of Release Rise & Shine Tea

1 (2-inch) piece fresh ginger, peeled and thinly sliced

4 cups of Distilled or Spring Water

½ cup of Bourbon

Honey

INSTRUCTIONS

Add fresh ginger to 4 cups of water in a pan. Bring to a boil and let boil for 2 minutes. Remove pan from heat.

Add Release Rise & Shine tea (Can add tea to empty tea bags or loose in pan). Let steep for 15 minutes.

Using a strainer (or remove tea bags) strain the tea. Add honey to taste and stir

Whisk in bourbon and serve hot or warm.

*OPTIONAL add a dash of cayenne pepper for an extra kick

Makes 6 servings

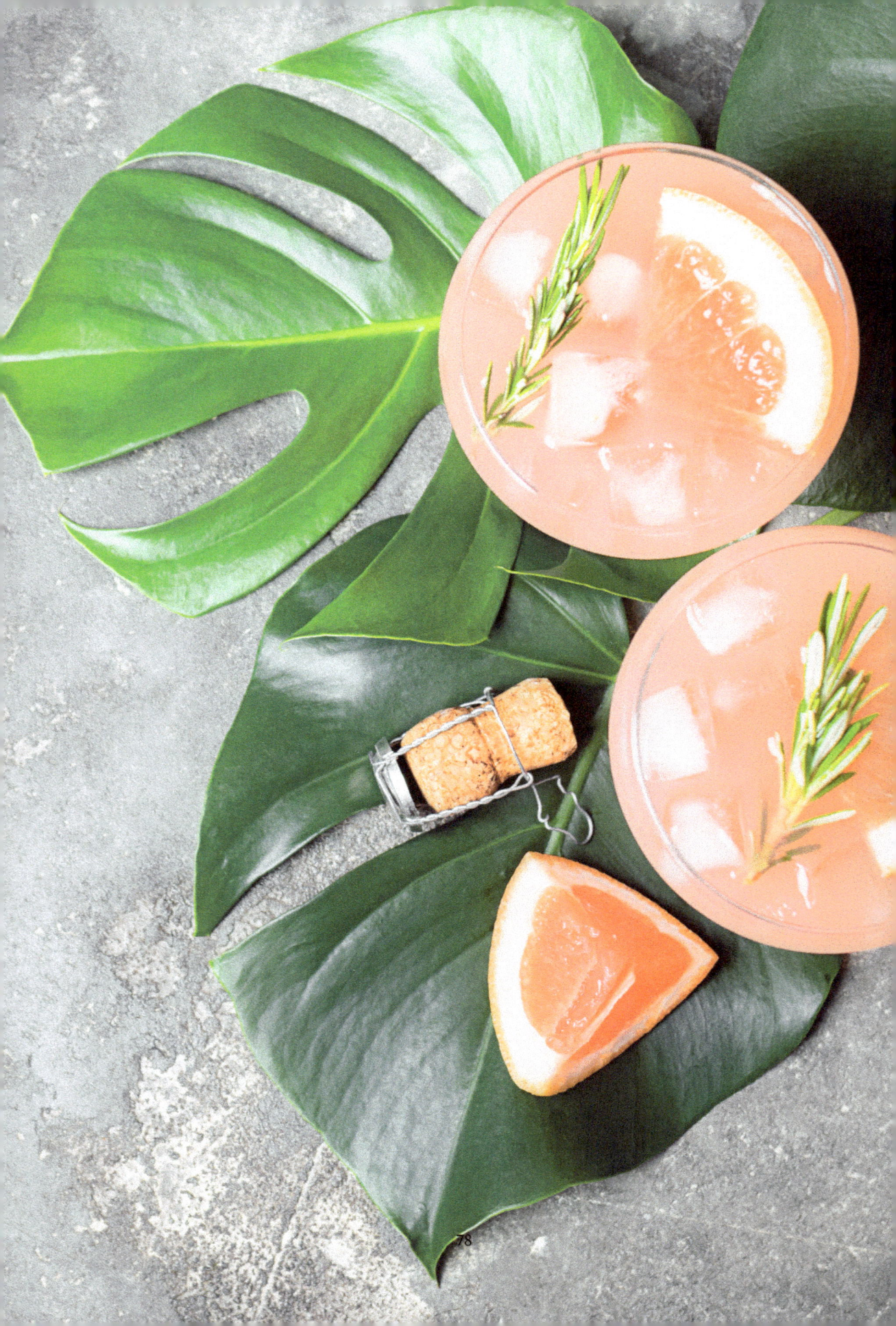

Pink Ginger Sunrise

INGREDIENTS

1 Tbsp. Release Rise & Shine Tea

10 oz. of Spring or Distilled Water

Juice of 1 Pink Grapefruit

½ cup of Ginger Beer

Honey to taste

INSTRUCTIONS

Bring water to a boil. Add 1 tablespoon of Release Rise & Shine tea to pot (can add tea to empty tea bags or loose in pan). Let steep for 7-10 minutes.

Using a strainer (or remove tea bags) strain the tea. Sweeten to taste with honey/agave etc.

Allow to cool. Chill in the refrigerator for at least 1 hour (this can be made ahead of time).

Once chilled, add grapefruit juice, stir and pour into ice-filled glasses

Top with ginger beer

OPTIONAL

To make this a G & G drink, add your favorite spirit such as rum or vodka

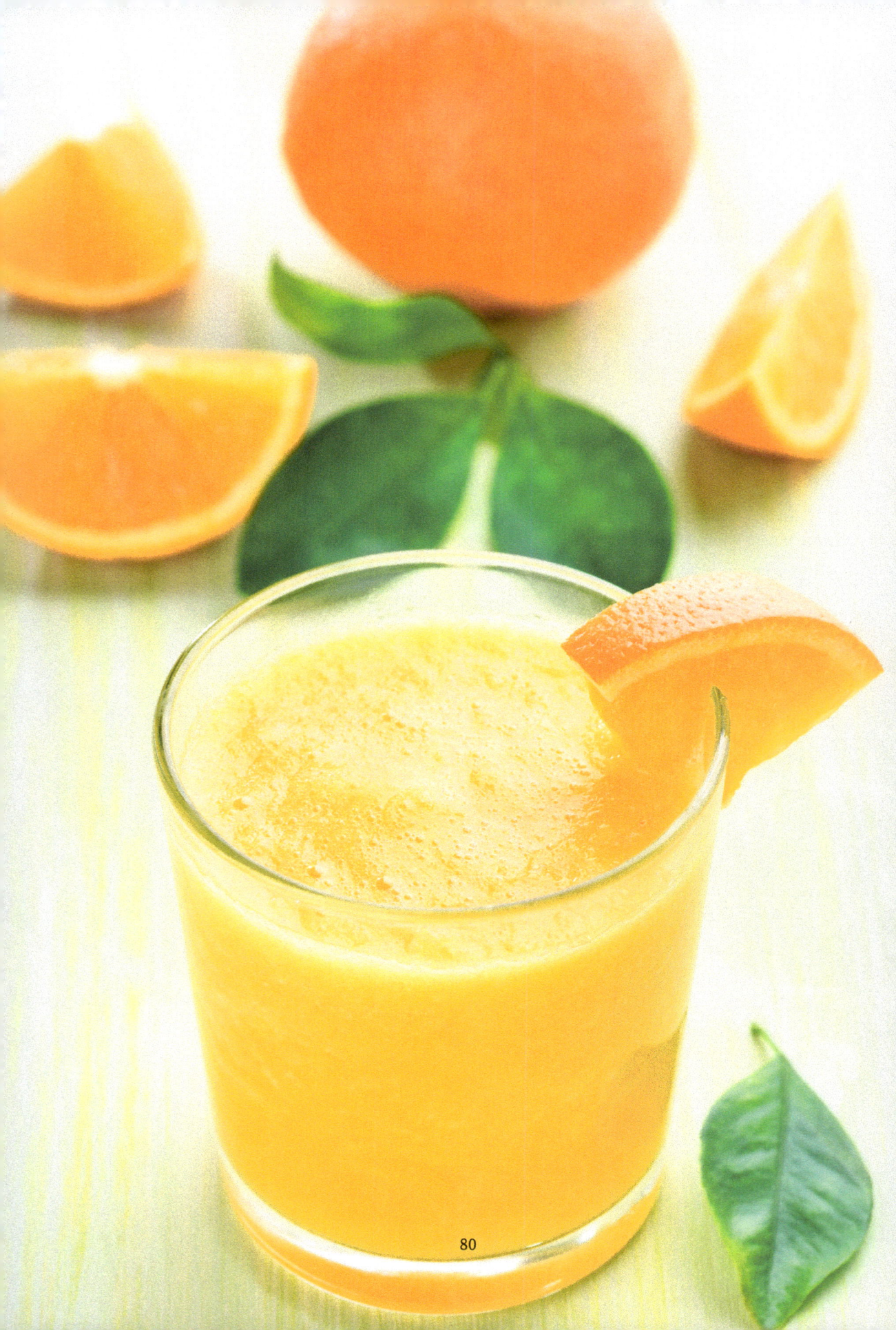

Sunshine Orange Smoothie

INGREDIENTS

1 Orange, peeled

1 tbsp. of Release Rise & Shine Tea

1 cup of Distilled or Spring Water

¼ Coconut Milk

2 Ice Cubes

1 tsp Vanilla Extract

Honey (optional)

INSTRUCTIONS

Boil water. Once boiled, add 1 tablespoon of Release Rise & Shine tea. Allow to steep for at least 5 minutes. Strain and allow to cool to at least room temperature.

Add peeled oranges split in sections, ice cubes, coconut milk and vanilla to a blender. Add brewed tea.

Blend until the oranges are completely smooth and your desired consistency.

May add honey to desired sweetness.

NOTES

*Make this smoothie to your taste. Can opt to add banana, strawberries or a little spinach for added nutritional value.

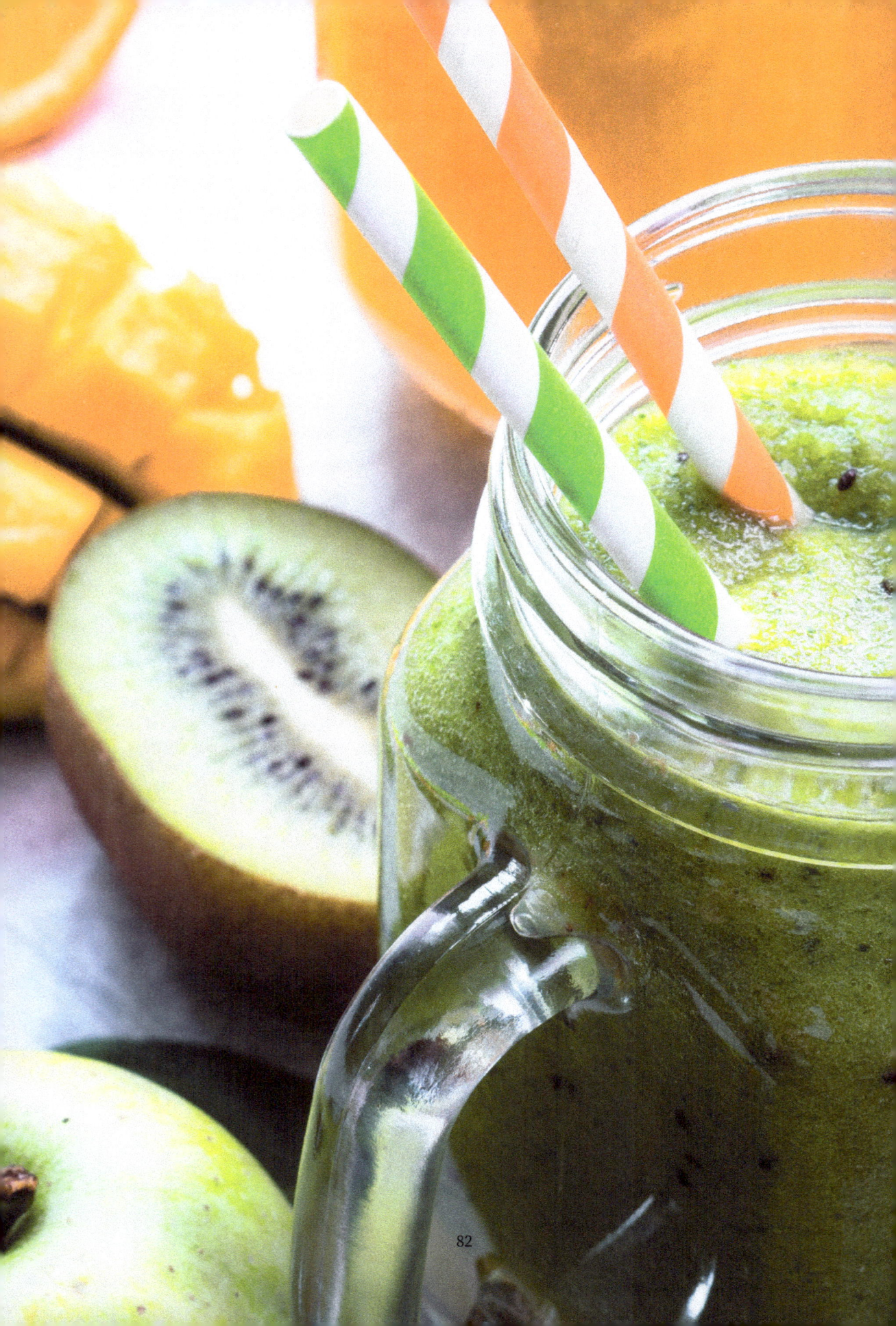

Release, Rise & Island Shine Smoothie

INGREDIENTS

1 ½ cup of Release, Rise & Shine tea, brewed

½ - ¾ cup Pineapple (in chunks)

½ Mango

INSTRUCTIONS

Add all ingredients in a blender

Blend until smooth

Add more tea or water, if necessary, to desired consistency

Optional add honey to taste

Chapter 7

Release Chill & Chai

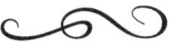

FREEALITEA's spin on chai tea was birthed in the fall of 2021. As the color of the leaves were changing, so were major changes occurring in my life. I had just packed up everything from my house in New Orleans, moved it to a storage unit in Atlanta, then went to my Daddy in Indianapolis to care for him as he was battling laryngeal (throat) cancer. I was a caregiver for my mother, godmother, and godfather so I was confident that I was prepared for how I needed to care for my father. I was wrong. It was one of the most difficult things I have done in life. I barely ate, got very little sleep, and literally put my whole life to include my business, plans, and personal wellness on hold and made him a priority. That way of being is not sustainable and my body and mind were feeling it. I was stressed, overwhelmed, exhausted, and needed something that warmed my soul and calmed my mind. A chai tea is something that reminds you of getting cozy as the temperatures get colder. I needed something to make me feel cozy and comforted. So, I put a FREEALITEA spin on a traditional chai and Release Chill & Chai was born!

I made myself sit down to sip it slowly as opposed to drinking on the go while preparing things for my Daddy. The flavors had depth that cascaded over me like my grandmother's afghan. I found a piece of peace and a 5-minute relaxing escape in the cup. I could sit back, release, and chill with this cup of chai.

Release Chill & Chai Ingredients:
- Black Tea
- Ginger Root
- Maca Root
- Cinnamon
- Cardamom
- Clove
- Allspice

Release Chill & Chai Benefits:

- Chai tea has antibacterial properties due to the presence of cinnamon, clove, and cardamom. They help prevent digestive issues caused by bacterial infections.

- Clove is a natural anti-inflammatory agent, as well as has natural anti-viral properties. This is a go-to for oral health. It can help prevent the overload of bacteria in the mouth, gingivitis and periodontal disease.

- Cardamom is helpful in lowering blood pressure. It is high in antioxidants and a natural diuretic which both contribute to lowering blood pressure.

Cardamom also improves oxygenation and breathing. Even diffusing the essential oil in aromatherapy will help improve the body's use of oxygen during exercise. Studies have shown that it improves breathing by helping bronchodilation (opening of airways) in the lungs.

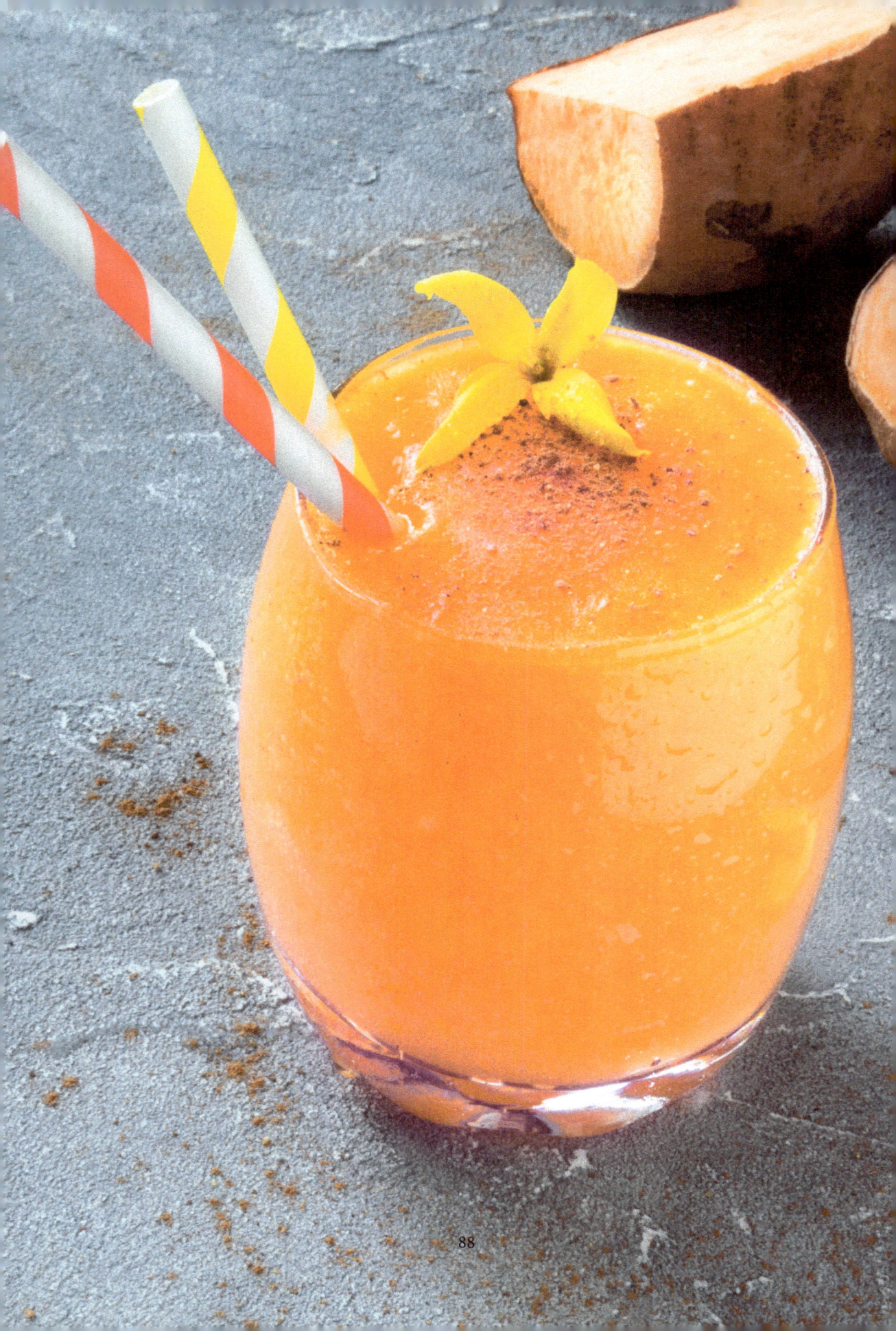

Chill & Chai Superfood Smoothie

I love this spin on a smoothie that provides extra vitamins and nutrients with the added cauliflower and sweet potato. Want to provide more veggies for those picky eaters? They'll never see this coming!

INGREDIENTS

1 tbsp. Release Chill & Chai simple syrup

½ small Sweet Potato diced, steamed and previously frozen

¼ cup Frozen Cauliflower

½ tsp Vanilla Extract

1 Medjool date, pitted

pinch of black pepper

1 ¼ cups unsweetened vanilla almond milk, cashew, oat or coconut milk (start with 1 cup and add the extra ¼ cup if necessary for desired consistency)

INSTRUCTIONS

Combine all ingredients in a high powdered blender and blend until super thick and creamy!

Optionally garnish with additional cinnamon, cardamom, and a sprinkle of hemp seeds. Enjoy immediately.

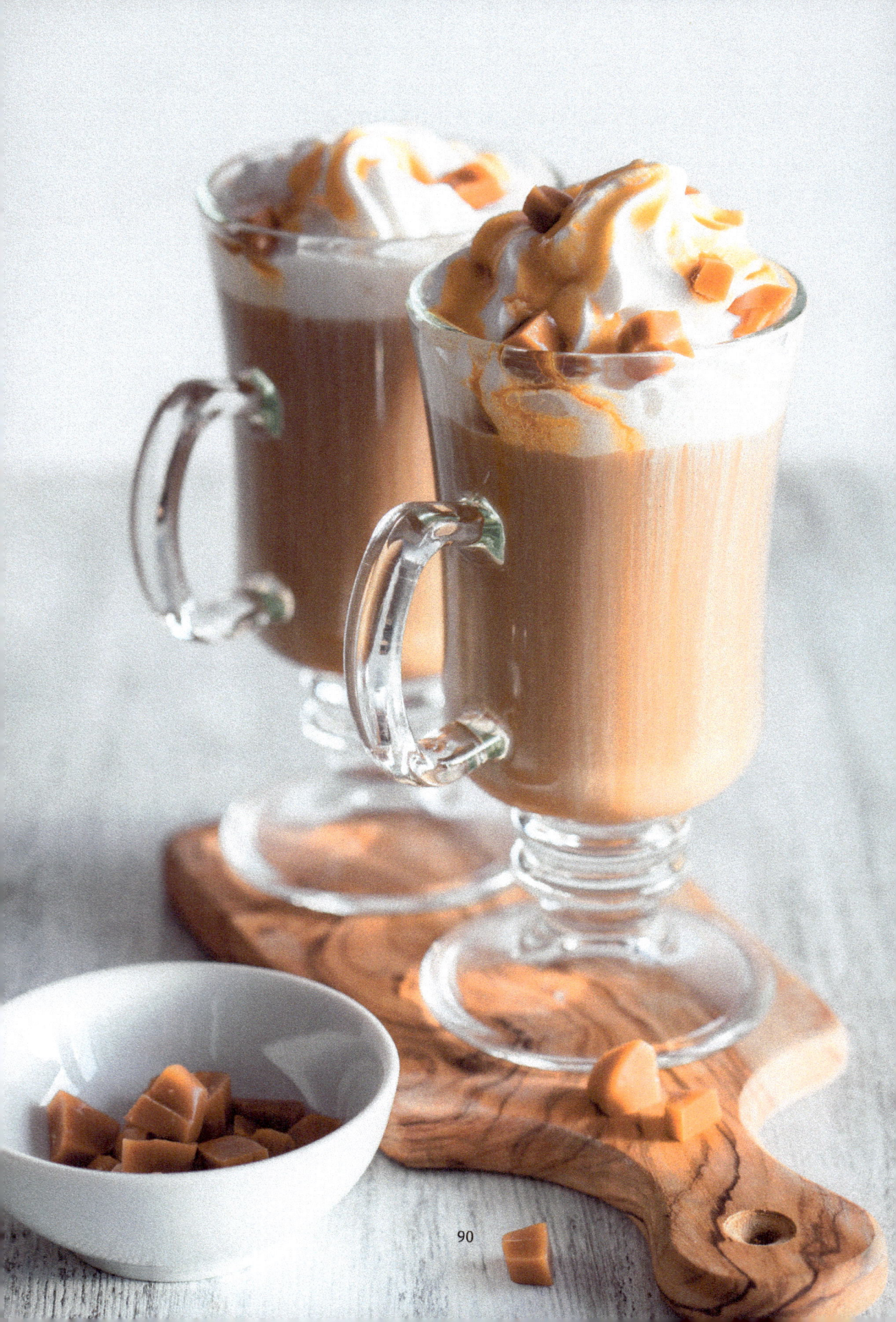

Salted Caramel Chill & Chai Latte

INGREDIENTS

2 tbsp Release Chill & Chai

2 cups milk (cashew, almond, oat, cow etc.), divided

1 tsp vanilla

For Garnish:

- Caramel Sauce
- Pinch of Sea Salt
- Whipped Cream

INSTRUCTIONS

In a medium saucepan heat 1 cup of milk to just before boiling. Turn off the heat. Add 2 tablespoons of Release Chill & Chai tea to an empty tea bag. Add tea to pot. Cover and allow to steep for 10 minutes.

Remove tea (strain or remove tea bag)

Add remaining ingredients to saucepan. Whisk together.

Heat the mixture over medium-high heat for 6-10 minutes or until the mixture is hot but not boiling.

To make the latte frothy, blend in a blender. Alternatively, may whisk vigorously while mixture is heating.

Drizzle caramel sauce on the inside of 4 glasses

After frothing, pour the finished latte mixture into 4 glasses

Top with whipped cream and drizzle with caramel sauce.

Top with a pinch of sea salt

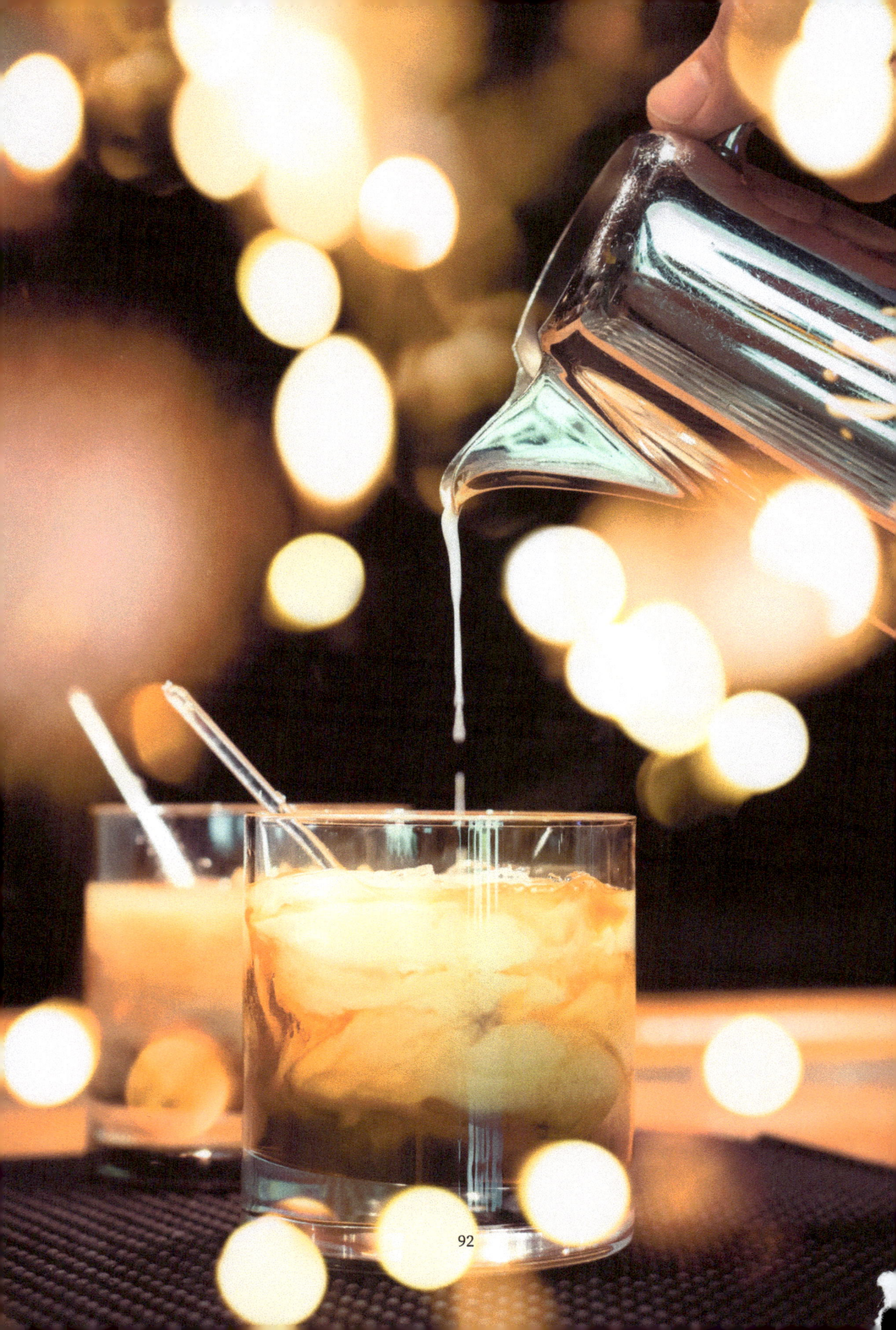

Chill & Chai White Russian

¼ cup Vodka

1 ½ ounces (3 tablespoons) Kahlua

1-2 ounces (2-4 tablespoons) Chill & Chai simple syrup

1-2 ounces (2-4 tablespoons) Heavy Cream or Milk of choice

Cinnamon Sticks and Star Anise, for garnish

INSTRUCTIONS

- Fill a glass with ice. Add the vodka, Kahlua, and Chill & Chai simple syrup. Stir gently.
- Add the heavy cream or milk and stir to combine.
- Garnish with a cinnamon stick and star anise, if desired.

ENJOY

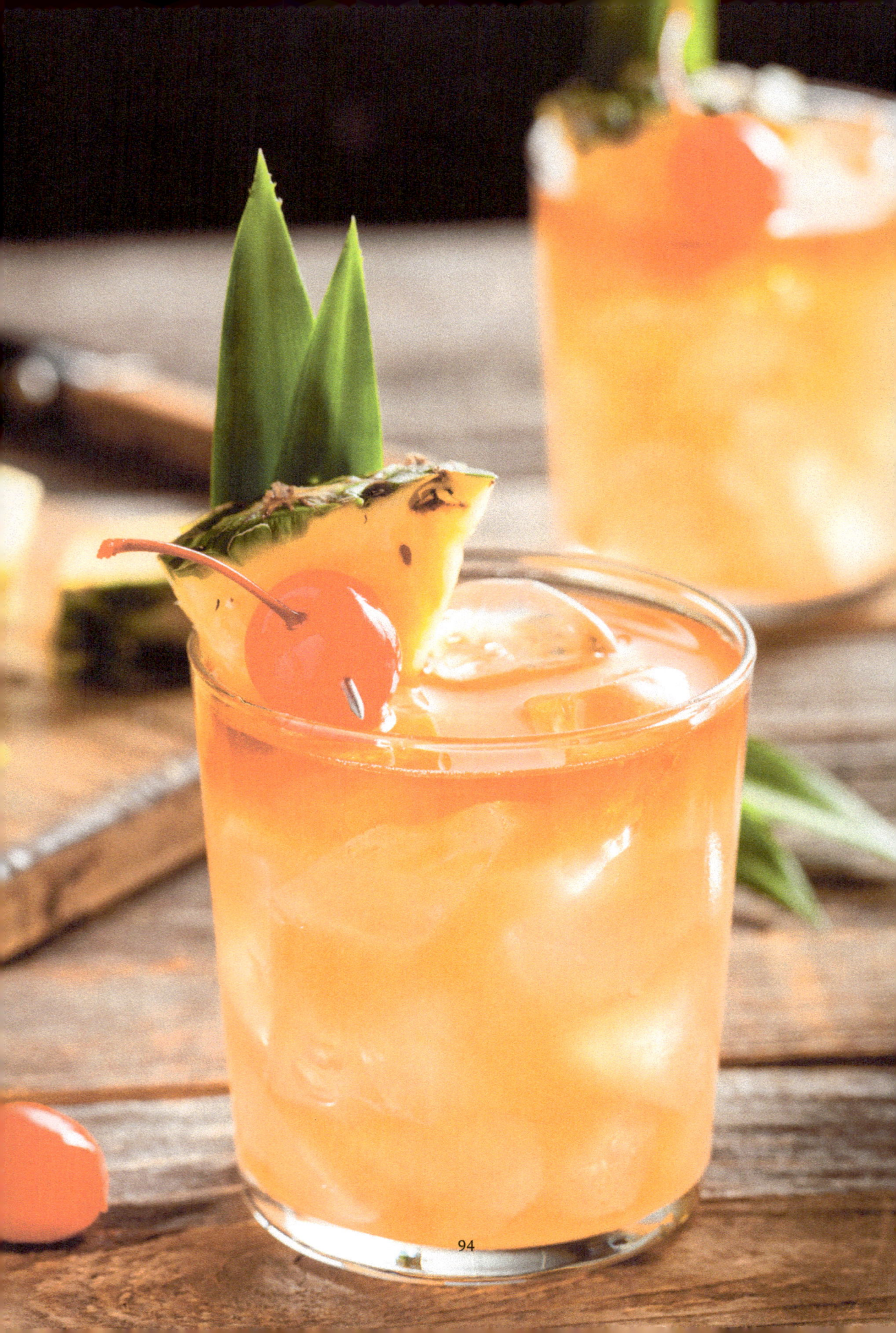

Chill with Chai & Tai

INGREDIENTS

2 oz. Dark Rum

2 tbsp Release Chill & Chai simple syrup

1 tbsp. Lemon juice

1 oz. Triple sec

1 tbsp. Grenadine

Pineapple Wedge or Orange Slice for garnish

INSTRUCTIONS

Blend rum, Chill & Chai simple syrup, lemon juice and triple sec in a shaker over ice.

Strain into a tall glass

Add a splash of grenadine.

Garnish with pineapple or orange slice

CHEERS!

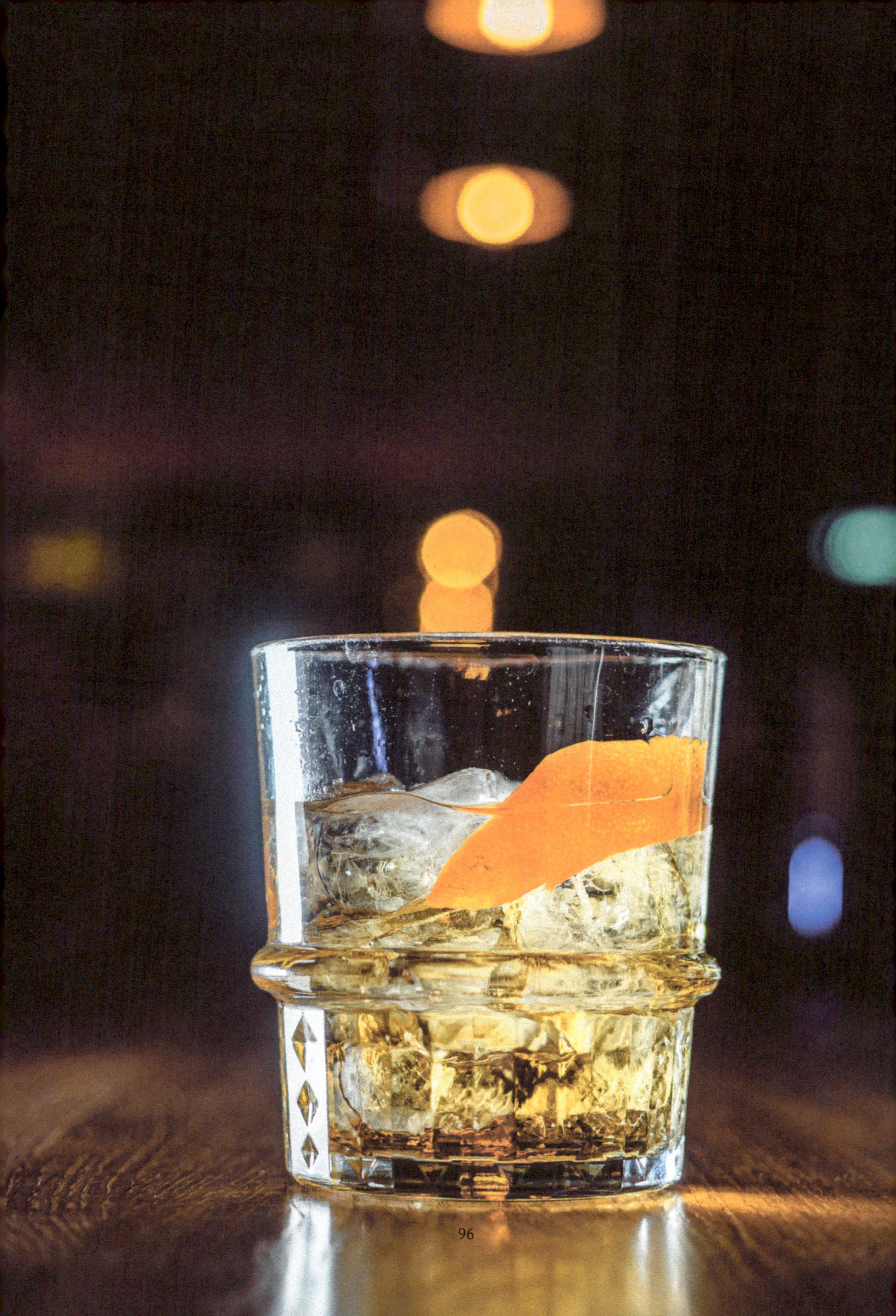

Chai Amaretto Punch

INGREDIENTS

2 tbsp Release Chill & Chai simple syrup

1 oz. Water

1 oz. Amaretto

2 oz. Vodka

Splash of Pineapple Juice

INSTRUCTIONS

Combine above ingredients and pour over ice.

Chapter 8

Sip Soothe & SensualiTEA

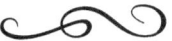

Have you ever been in so much emotional pain and overwhelmed that you went numb? A feeling like the old school movie, "Invasion of the Body-snatchers", but your soul was snatched?

Honey, been there done that!

In an ever-changing world full of uncertainty amid an over-extended life, most of us are running like three blind mice. We are disconnected from our feelings, emotions, and the moment. We're always thinking about what needs to be done, what's next etc.

It wasn't until after I ended a 7 ½ year relationship and he finally moved all his items out that I was left to deal with myself. I realized I had flicked the switch off to my feelings. Sometimes it seemed easier not to feel, than to feel pain and disappointment. It left me feeling hollow and lifeless, almost like a zombie.

In March of 2022, I had reiki for the first time. For those of you not familiar with reiki, it is a healing energy technique that promotes relaxation, reduces stress, and aids in becoming energetically balanced physically, emotionally, mentally, and spiritually. Some refer to it as a body energy modality just like acupuncture, qigong, reflexology, and EFT (Emotional Freedom Technique). The word reiki is made up of two Japanese words. Rei meaning, "God's wisdom" and ki meaning "vital life force energy. Therefore, reiki is," spiritually guided life-force energy." Most of the time a reiki practitioner doesn't touch you or may use light touch.

During my reiki session, I felt the sensation of a stone in my chest cavity right below my sternum where an open and loving heart used to be. It isn't something that I had ever felt before, but it was a message for me that my heart had grown cold. That was a surprise to me because I always thought of myself as a very loving and caring person.

One day I was getting a massage and just started crying uncontrollably; you know the ugly cry. This woman with healing and magical hands, started awakening my senses. I began to feel again.

As the switch of my senses went from dark to dim, I realized not only had I blocked the feelings of disappointment and pain, but also pleasure and delight.

Thus began a journey of deeper understanding of myself and self-discovery. For me that meant a lot of quiet time of reflection, meditation, and consistent sessions with my therapist.

I came to my senses and started doing the work to feel again and engage each and every one of my senses – taste, touch, smell, hearing, and sight.

My mind started to open, my heart started feeling hopeful, my lady parts started tingling, and my mood AND libido were lifted. I started feeling like a desirable woman again. Coming to my senses led to FEELING again. And not just feeling, but sensual, sexual, empowered, and FREE!

I sipped FREEALTEA and allowed it to soothe my soul then my body followed. I sought to experience pleasure every day by bringing joy and bliss to one of my five senses. Pleasure is not confined to the bedroom, it's something that can be experienced every day in any moment; to living fully in the blessings and bliss in life!

It's about experiencing the moment

Being in the moment

Creating the moment

I did that by engaging all my senses and fully feeling and experiencing them.

Next, I created physical sensual experiences for myself that I coined, "M & M". What is M & M you ask? It is meditation and masturbation.

I had long ago dismissed the idea of what brought me pleasure.

Dr. Ben said, "Heaven lies between a Black woman's thighs." While meditating to be in tune and at one with my DIVINE self, find my calm, and receive DIVINE messages; I touched my heaven learning myself and exploring myself in an intimate way. Sensations I hadn't felt in years were awakened and ignited. As I climaxed, I released, took a large exhale and breathed out pent up fears and frustrations. Then just basked in the energetic life force and allowed it to diffuse throughout my body and psyche. The M & M became a powerful force that calmed my mind and elevated my energy. I felt like a powerful GODDESS! I was light and lifted!

As a result of a deeper level of intimacy (into-me-see), a Sip Soothe & SensualiTEA blend was born – FREEALITEA's Sensual Blend.

This tea is great for libido, menopause symptoms such as hot flashes, and balancing hormones.

Sensual Blend Ingredients:

- ❁ Horny Goat Weed
- ❁ Damiana
- ❁ Maca Root
- ❁ Cinnamon
- ❁ Cacao Nibs
- ❁ Rose Petals

- ❄ Honey Granules
- ❄ Dark Chocolate Cocoa Powder

Sensual Blend Benefits:

- Damiana is an herb that feels like a goddess to me. From the time you smell her, you feel warmth in your soul. She helps bring your inner goddess forth. The leaves lift the mood by reducing stress, as well as lifting the libido. Damiana increases blood flow, particularly to the pelvic area which increases sensitivity and heightens stimulation.

- Maca Root is also known as Peruvian Ginseng because of its ability to increase energy and stamina but it also decreases stress. Because of its ability to balance the hormones estrogen, progesterone, and testosterone, it is a go to for my seasoned ladies experiencing perimenopause symptoms. Studies show that maca root can help improve sexual desire and sexual dysfunction in women. Fellas can benefit as well by helping to balance testosterone. Testosterone decreases in all of us as we age.

- Horny Goat Weed is an herb used in Traditional Chinese Medicine. It can increase blood flow to small vessels thereby helping to increase libido and energy. Some of its other uses are:

- Hypertension

- Hay Fever

- Menopause symptoms

Since it has a stimulating effect, use caution if taking blood pressure medications, have thyroid disease, or a hormone sensitive cancer.

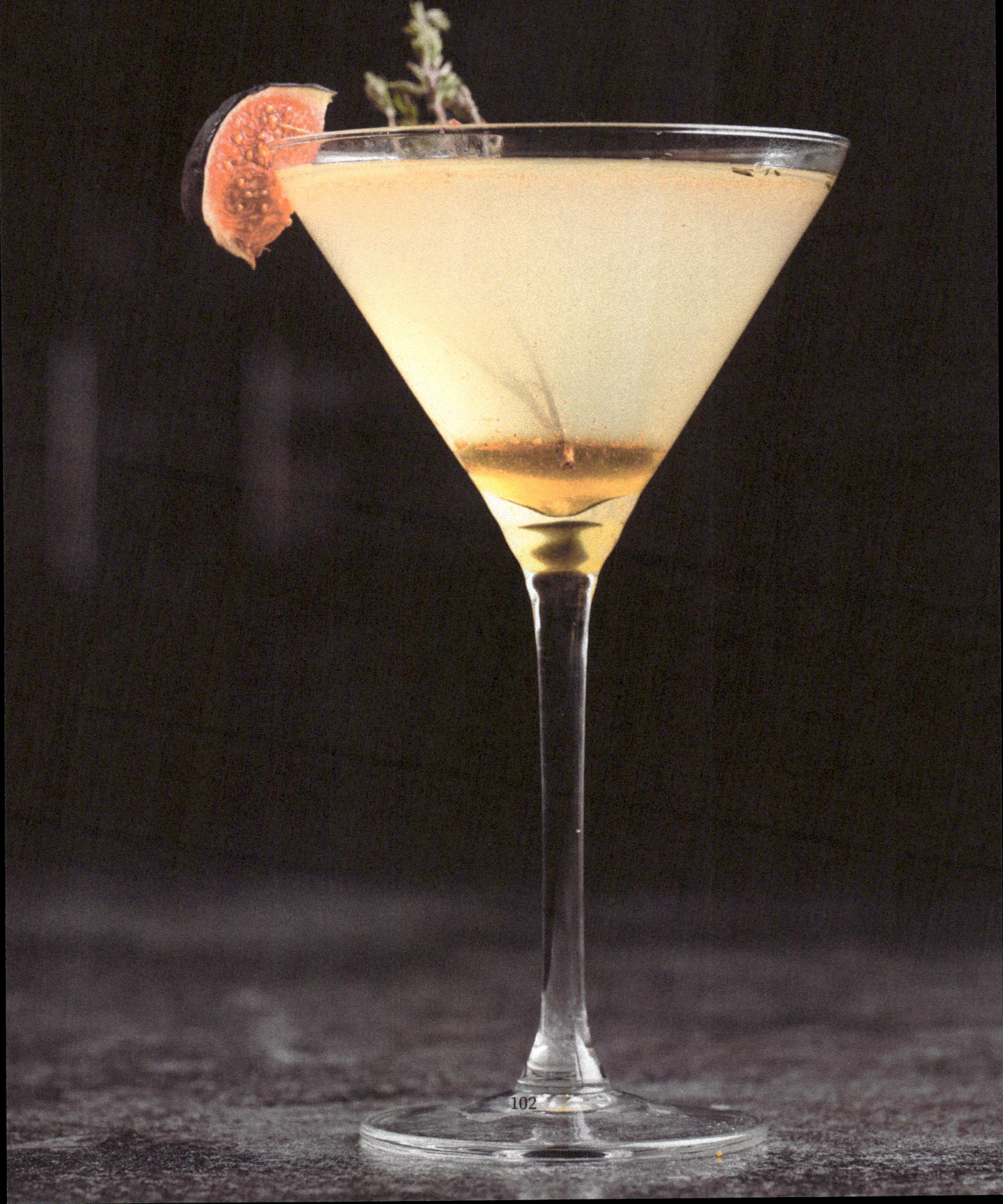

BUTTER BABY

INGREDIENTS

1 tablespoon FREEALITEA's Sensual Blend

1 oz. Vodka

1 oz. Caribbean Rum

1 tablespoon Butter

Honey (to taste)

INSTRUCTIONS

Bring 10 oz. of water to a boil. Add 1 tablespoon of FREEALITEA's Sensual Blend. Allow to steep for 5-7 minutes. Strain. Melt the butter and mix it with the honey.

Add the brewed tea.

Pour equal parts into 2 cocktail glasses.

Add an equal amount of rum and vodka.

Stir and ENJOY!

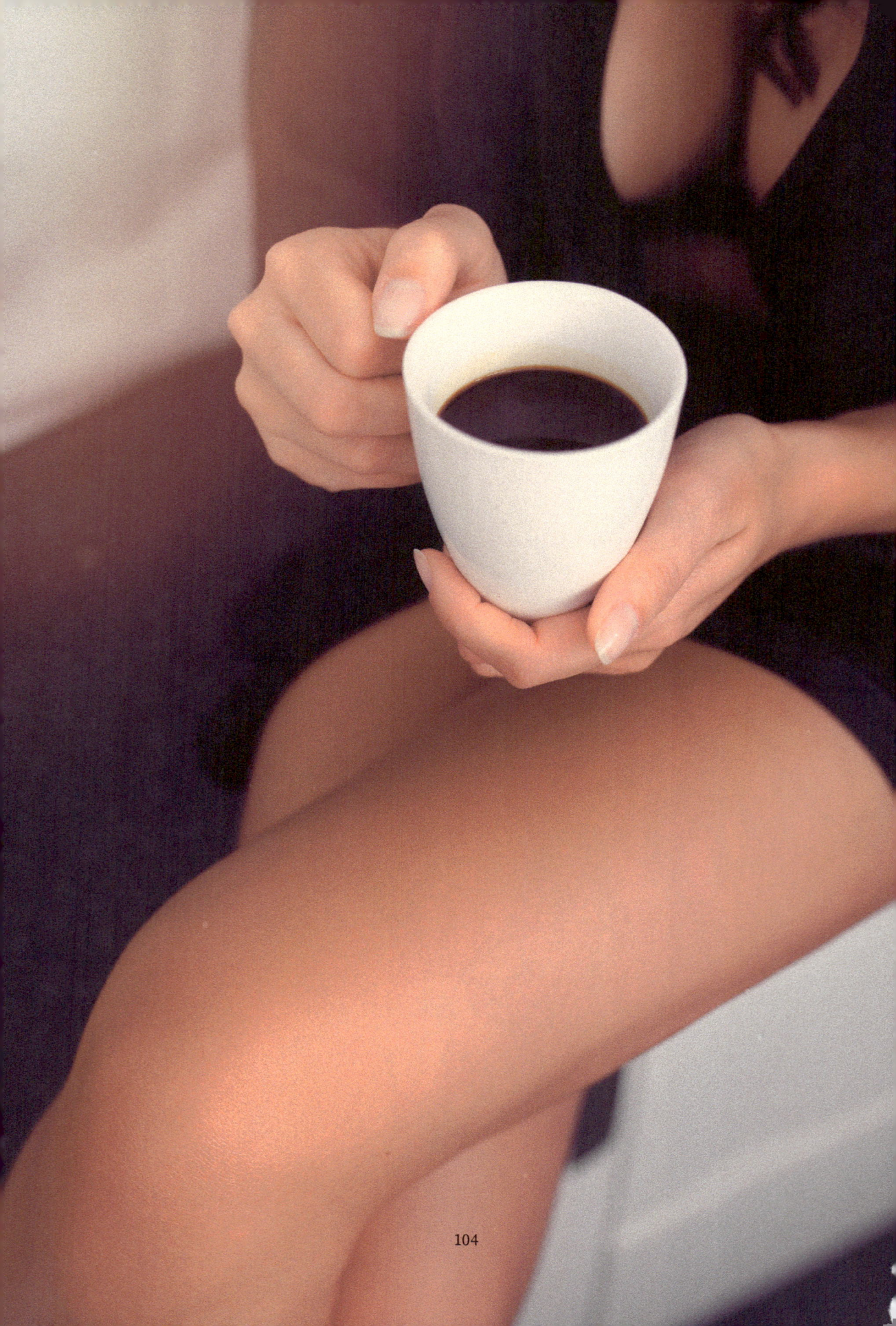

SENSUAL CHOCOLATE ZEN

INGREDIENTS

1 tbsp FREEALITEA's Sensual Blend

½ cup Organic Coconut Milk (canned version) + ½ cup Water (or 1 cup any non-dairy milk)

Pinch of Pink Salt

Honey to taste

½ tsp Vanilla Extract (optional)

INSTRUCTIONS

Bring ½ cup of water to a boil.

Add 1 tablespoon of FREEALITEA's Sensual blend. Allow to steep for 5-7 minutes.

Warm coconut milk (not to a boiling point). Once warmed, add to Sensual tea.

Stir in pinch of Himalayan Pink Salt, vanilla extract and honey.

ENJOY!

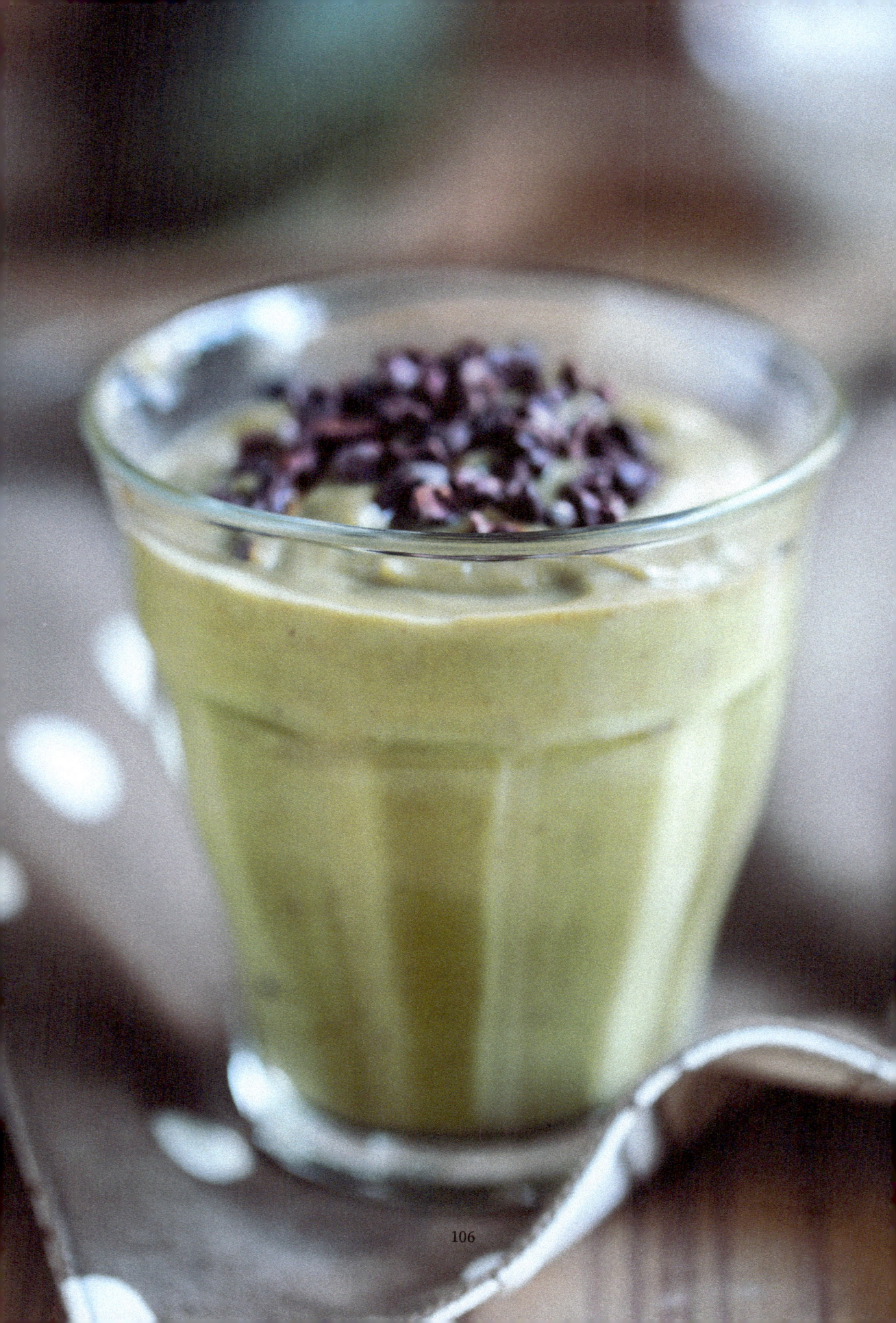

Green Aphrodisiac Smoothie

INGREDIENTS

2 tbsp. FREEALITEA's Sensual Blend

1 cup Milk (coconut, cashew, almond. or oat. Your choice)

1 cup Fresh Water

3 Medjool Dates

¼ Avocado

1/3 cup of Spinach

1 tsp Raw Honey

Small piece of Ginger Root

½ tsp Vanilla Extract

Cayenne Pepper (optional)

INSTRUCTIONS

Bring 1 cup of water to a boil. Add the Sensual Blend tea (Can add tea to empty tea bags or loose in pan). Let steep for 7 minutes. Using a strainer (or remove tea bags) strain the tea. Set to the side and allow to cool.

Soak Medjool dates in water overnight for easier blending.

In a high-powered blender, add milk then ginger root. Allow the ginger to blend completely. Add remaining ingredients to blender.

Blend until smooth

Pour into two different glasses.

Optionally add a dash of cayenne pepper for an extra hit.

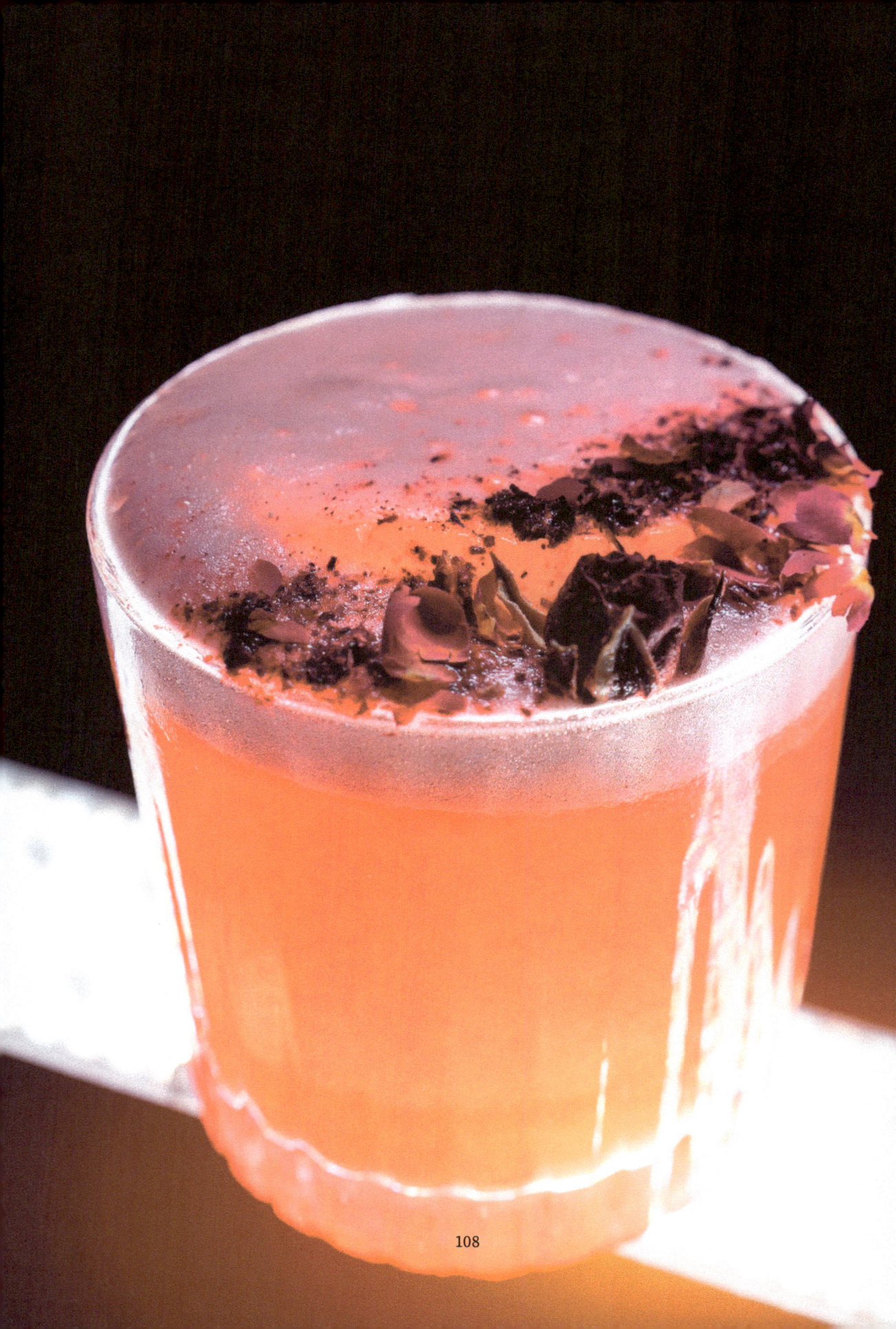

For Goddess Sake

INGREDIENTS

1 tbsp. FREEALITEA'S Sensual Blend

3 ounces dry sake

Handful of Raspberries

1 spritz Rosewater

INSTRUCTIONS

Place the Sensual Blend in an empty teabag. Place teabag in a glass air-tight container such as a mason jar. Add sake and allow it to cold steep for 8 hours.

Gently squeeze tea bag when removing.

Muddle with fresh raspberries, shake with ice and pour over a cocktail strainer into a chilled cup or martini glass. Garnish with raspberries and spritz with rose water.

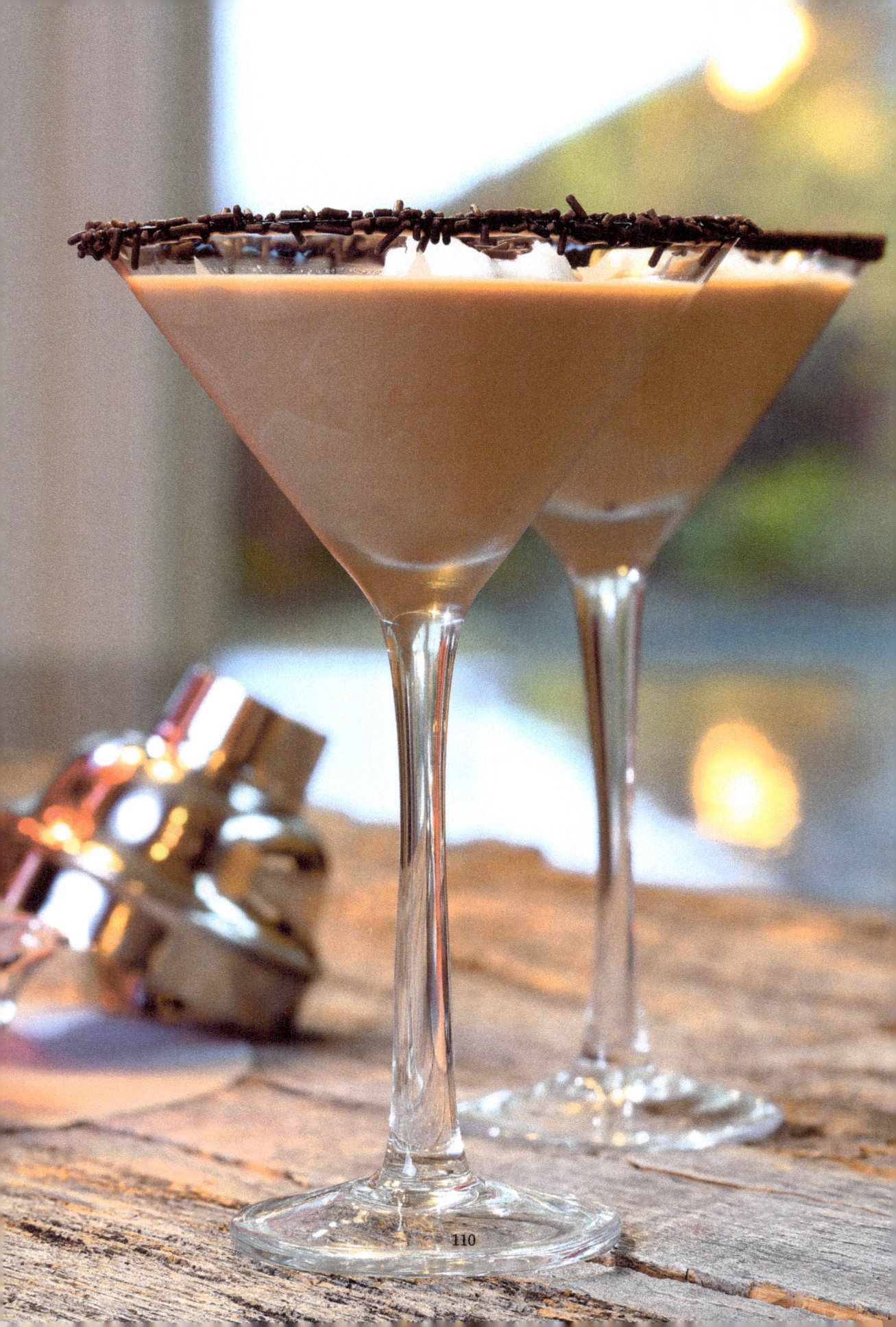

Chocolate SensualiTEAni

INGREDIENTS

1 cup dark chocolate chips

2 cups coconut milk

1 pinch sea salt

½ Tbsp Sensual Blend simple syrup

Chocolate Sauce (garnish)

Chocolate Sprinkles (garnish)

INSTRUCTIONS

Add the coconut milk to a small pot and bring to a boil over medium heat. Turn off the stove and remove the pot from the heat right as it boils.

Add the chocolate chips and salt to the pot and stir with a whisk. Keep stirring until the chocolate chips have completely melted and are blended into the milk.

Add Sensual Blend simple syrup and stir.

Pour the chocolate martini mix into a bowl or pitcher, cover and refrigerate.

Pour some chocolate syrup on a shallow plate and put the sprinkles on a separate plate.

Dip the rim on a martini glass in the chocolate syrup and then into the sprinkles.

Use a whisk to give the chocolate martini mocktail mix a stir.

Pour chocolate mix into each prepared martini glass.

Enjoy chilled!

*NOTE To make the G & G (good & grown) version, add vodka.

CONCLUSION

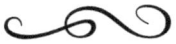

I dedicate this book to the four people in my life that always made me feel safe to fully express myself: to fully and unapologetically be myself without judgement.

That is my grandmother affectionately known as "Nanny", my mother affectionately known as "Palie", my brother affectionately known as "Head", and the love of my life affectionately known as "Honey Baby".

With them I always felt seen, heard, and loved. With them I've always felt safe to express, explore, and engage ALL my senses. A daily ritual of sipping with FREEALITEA and allowing my senses and DIVINE self to be elevated is what attracted this beautiful King Man into my life! Thank you, Honey Baby, for covering me and creating a safe place for me to fully be me in ALL my Michelleisms!

From their loving touch to their listening ear, I've been FREE to be me and create my own reality!

I pray recipes and messages in this book will help you do the same.

Be well!

Dr. Michelle

www.freealitea.com

www.ingramcontent.com/pod-product-compliance
Lightning Source LLC
Chambersburg PA
CBHW041119120626
46547CB00019B/2764